My Journey to the Fountain of Youth

(A Journey Through the Internet to Look and Feel Years Younger)

By Christopher Welch Gault

———————————————————

May you find your inner strength to achieve all that you dream.

Do you want to look years younger as you age? Who in their right mind wouldn't? This amazing journey took me through the Internet to find the very best solutions to aging well, also known as anti-aging. Grow your hair back or thicker and healthier, get rid of wrinkles and improve skin quality, get in fantastic shape by building muscle and losing fat, eat healthier, get your mind right and learn to live a happier, healthier and fuller life. You won't regret purchasing this book!

Note from Author to Those Purchasing the Paperback

If you purchased the paperback version of this book you should take advantage of the obtaining the free kindle version as well (free to those who purchase the paperback). There are many links to other websites and videos in this book and the kindle version will facilitate that process.

Table of Contents

Chapter 1 – Introduction

So, when I was in my mid-fifties, I noticed that I seemed to be aging faster than I should – losing almost all my hair and noticing many wrinkles on my face, neck and hands. I found it harder to complete my workouts (I have always been active) and found myself getting hurt more often and taking longer to recover.

In contrast to this, I noticed many people my age seemed to appear a lot younger than their chronological age. They were more active and seemed to be living happier, healthier lives than most others. But I did notice others that were living lives quite the opposite. They were my age but looked as if they could be my parents. They typically weren't happy and, I hate to use the words, really let themselves go and fell into a hopeless deep hole on the dark side of life.

Why was this? I pondered on it for a long time. I mean, how come some people were living great, very positive lives and others were aging faster than they should and becoming more and more bitter towards others and the world in general? I mean I was pretty active and my diet wasn't bad, but something was missing. Because of this, I asked myself a question: *Do you want to feel and look years younger?* Actually, when I thought about it, that's a bit of a silly question. I mean who in their right mind wouldn't? Then I asked the correct question: *Was I willing to do the research and work to look and feel years younger?*

I had to ask myself the question again because the answer was not that easy. Did I have the time? Did I have the motivation? Was I willing to make the commitment? Where do I even start?

Should I put a good amount of time into this? I came back with a solid maybe. At least I would give it my best shot.

But how to even start to become healthier and younger both physically and mentally? I really didn't have a clue. As I mentioned before, I was always active, worked out, and watched my diet (or at least I thought I did) so what was the problem? The people I mentioned that looked very young for their age were muscular, had low body fat and their skin just radiated with youth. What was their secret and how come I didn't know it? How come some people aged gracefully and others didn't? Was it all predetermined by good vs. bad genes or was there a way to modify one's lifestyle and take control of their own destiny?

I must admit that I am a big fan of controlling my own destiny. So, when I came to that part of the debate playing out In my mind (destiny vs. fate) I decided to give this *aging well* lifestyle a go – and I mean really give it an honest attempt!

After all, there are mainly two types of people in the world. Those that blame their predicament on everything and everyone other than themselves and those that take the responsibility to control their own happiness and fate. Which of these two do you suppose enjoys life more?

With all that said, this book will go over my personal journey to feel and look better as I age. As I proceeded through my journey, and it is still going on, I learned good and bad news when it comes to re-growing my hair (as I mentioned earlier, I went bald early in my life), reducing wrinkles from my face, toning and putting on muscle on my body, increasing the health of every cell in my body, getting my mind right and generally looking and feeling years younger.

Basically *aging well*, which I like that term better than *anti-aging*. Anti-aging means you don't age – basically you are dead. We all age, we can't stop time, but it's how we age. We can either age well or age not so well. I chose aging well!

The good news is that I found out that it's very possible to achieve these goals and it can be done naturally and doesn't have to be expensive. Now, that's the good news. The bad news (although I don't like saying *bad*) I learned, is that it takes patience, time and effort. But it will work – you just have to put in the time and work and you have to be consistent.

I just want to take a moment to say that I did take care of my body pretty much my whole life, but I wasn't perfect. I also neglected good facial and hair health. Because of that, even though my body was nice and toned (although not perfect) my face became wrinkled and my hair fell out. Actually, spending a lot of time in the sun (without sunscreen) my face became old fast. I also started balding in my twenties and by the time I started down the road to the *Fountain of Youth* I was completely bald on the top of my head.

Not a pretty sight.

Yes, I was aging quickly. But not anymore. I fixed that. And so can anyone who is willing to put the time in to get their youthful life back. I mean we all have the choice to either experience accelerated aging – get wrinkly, balding, flabby, cranky, mean and grey or we can take charge of our life and change it for the better.

I chose to take charge of my life and make it better.

One thing I did know was in order to change I had to change something. What I'm saying is even though life has selected a physical and mental path for us, we can change that predetermined path and take control of our lives. But it takes changing what we do, and it takes work. Obviously doing what I was doing wasn't getting the job done. What was the definition of insanity again? Doing the same thing over and over again and hoping for different results? Basically if you want to change for the better, you have to make changes to your daily life. Change doesn't occur automatically.

So we can do what we have always done and let time get the best of us or we can chose to make a change for the better. The good thing is it's up to us. The only caveat is that we must take control of our lives to make the changes happen.

Don't believe me? Here is one example of an individual who didn't accept his situation and changed his life drastically: There was a skinny boy from Austria who came from an impoverished environment. His father was a police officer and so was his brother. He basically had a path laid out in front of him that he didn't want to accept. Basically, his environment limited him in what he could achieve, but that didn't stop this determined young individual.

This skinny adolescent developed a love for sports and fitness and against his father's wishes started working out with weights at age fifteen, ate healthy and had a positive attitude that he could attain anything that life had to offer. Basically, grasp the world with his hands and take it.

This scrawny child went on to win the Mr. Olympia body building contest as well as becoming a blockbuster Hollywood actor and the Governor of California. Obviously, I'm talking about Arnold Schwarzenegger. Now, do you think he would have accomplished a fraction of what he did if he just sat around the house eating bonbons? Of course not! It took a lot of hard work, dedication and the desire to change his life. The same holds true to looking and feeling years younger. It doesn't cost a lot but it does take patience, time and some good old fashion work.

By the way, Arnold, if I am lucky enough for you to read this, I apologize for the scrawny comment. Please, I beg you, don't beat the heck out of me!

So as I travelled down the Internet I was able to grow my hair back. I can tell you my new hair was not from a hair transplant, or toupee or any drug consisting of toxic chemicals that costs a fortune that I would have to take my entire lifetime. I was also able to reduce some wrinkles and it didn't take plastic surgery or Botox injections. So how did I shave years off my life without resorting to those conventional options?

I'm going to let you in on the secrets of how I accomplished my transformation and got my life back on track. But first a disclaimer. I am not an expert on any of the procedures or products that I'm going to share with you. I'm not a doctor nor a hair expert, chemist or biologist. I'm just going to inform you about my personal journey through the wealth of information that is available to anyone searching on the Internet that helped me get to where I am today.

So, if I'm not an expert why did you purchase the book? Is that what you're asking? Believe me, if you are serious about looking and feeling years younger, this is the best book you will ever read.

What I can help you do is cut through all the garbage that's out on the Internet (and other media) and show you what really works. How do I know this? Because I've gone through and investigated and tested these techniques and found out which ones worked, and which ones didn't.

With that said it doesn't mean that if I didn't include someone's website, videos or words of wisdom that they won't work as well but what I can say (and feel good about it) is what I share with you did work for me.

And I believe that's worth something!

I would also suggest that after you read this book and check out all the great Internet content I will share with you, that you continue to investigate healthy living topics yourself. As you know there is always new and improved content on the Internet every day. This book is just a start on the journey to *The Fountain of Youth*. I hope it inspires you to branch out and even come up with your own solutions that may work for you and others. After all, helping out others is one of the greatest gifts we can achieve.

At this point I want to mention that if you have a certain section you want to jump to then, by all means, jump to it. You won't hurt my feelings. I actually won't even know. I would hope that you will eventually read the whole book because I think there's some good stuff in here (I'm a little biased) but if you are losing your hair (or already lost it) and want to start curing that problem right away then feel free to jump to that section.

I also want to mention that I'm not going to bore you with all the science behind the techniques I'll share with you in this book. Don't get me wrong, I'll touch on the basics and I will direct you to where you can find as much science as you want to on the Internet, but I'm going to let the experts fill you in on all the details.

To further a point from the paragraph above, I just want to make sure that you all know that the individuals who have websites, Youtube channels and e-books that reveal these secrets have my upmost gratitude and respect since if it were not for them, I would not be on my own journey to find health, happiness and youth and this book would never have been written.

It should also be stated, so I'll go ahead and state it, that as you go through the book, please make sure to click on the links I reference and watch the videos and read the articles. This book was meant to go hand in hand with what I found on the Internet so please make sure to do that.

Even though this book has only 112 pages, the content is much greater. If you click on the links to the videos and articles, is much larger than the 112 pages. The kindle version is also easier because clicking on the links will take you to that content (as long as you have Internet access) so if you have the paperback, you may also want to invest in the kindle version. There is a great deal on amazon if to get the kindle book if you purchased the paperback.

So, read the book and go forth and get back those years you lost. You will be grateful you did! You can definitely get those years back and amaze your family and friends. And most of all, and more importantly, you will amaze and please yourself!

Chapter 2 – A quick note on basic health

So, before I reveal the details of my journey to *The Fountain of Youth* through the Internet, I just want to mention, and I realize this is common sense but it must be pointed out anyway – I was not going to appear and feel younger than my age if I ate garbage. So, if I was really interested in looking and feeling years younger, then I had to change my diet drastically. That pretty much meant I couldn't eat fast food ever again. Or, at best, very infrequently. And when I say infrequent I mean maybe once or twice a year (yes you heard that right).

I made a conscious effort to eat as much organic food as possible and I stayed away from preservatives, antibiotics, added hormones & steroids and bad carbohydrates (gluten, bleached & processed).

Basically, I had to eat healthy foods. After all, you are what you eat so I had to make a decision. What did I want my body, face and hair to look like: An old pile of garbage or the physique of a stunning movie star (not that I'm there but I strive to be)? It's totally up to us. We can make that decision, but we are also responsible for that decision. I know that sounds harsh and you probably just threw the book or your tablet on the floor never to pick it up again, but it is true. More on this later.

Before I move on, I feel compelled to say that one of the most important changes I made in my diet was to get rid of anything that had chemicals in it. So yes, that meant sodas, processed foods and any ingredient that an average ten-year-old can't pronounce.

I came by this interesting article in the Washington Post that lists how there are 19 ingredients in McDonald French fries: *There are 19 ingredients in McDonald's French fries* by Roberto A. Ferdman: https://www.washingtonpost.com/news/wonk/wp/2015/01/22/there-are-19-ingredients-in-mcdonalds-french-fries/?utm_term=.51cb6a7eb577. So, yes, McDonald's French fries have nearly twenty ingredients. Yes, I just said nearly twenty ingredients. To be healthy, I would think it should just be three. Potatoes, peanut oil (better yet unrefined coconut oil or baked) and Himalayan sea salt – and all the ingredients should be organic.

Nearly twenty ingredients! What the heck is in those fries? And from the article you can see that some of these ingredients sound like they are part of a disturbing chemistry lab experiment. I mean do we really need *Dimethylpolysiloxane* in our diets? Do we really want this anti-foaming agent in our bodies – our temples? Do we know the physical and mental effects of this chemical? Do vegetarians know that there is natural beef flavor in the french fries? What's TBHQ? Is this preservative harmful to our bodies? What are the long-term side effects of consuming these chemicals? Do you want to be the one who finds out? Better to let someone else be the guinea pig in this crazy experiment.

Let me ask you a question. Did you ever find some McDonald's french fries under the seat of your car a few months after you purchased them? Did you notice the french fries look exactly the same as they did when you purchased them months ago? Does anyone think that's normal?

The same can be said for McDonald's hamburgers. Don't believe me? Go buy one (please don't eat it) and put it on your desk and leave it there for a month or two. I guarantee it won't look much different from the day you purchased it. I don't know about you but I would stay away from that mess. I mean how many preservatives could possibly be in that hamburger to have it stay like new over that extensive period of time?

Scary!

Try the same experiment with a hamburger made from organic meat. It won't look the same. Just try it and you will see. It decays and becomes moldy because it's *real* food and not loaded with destructive chemicals.

Anyway, the moral of this story regarding this part of my journey is that I had to know what I was putting in my mouth and body and I needed to make wise, or at lease wiser, choices.

I have been approached by many who say they get tempted and can't help themselves – the cookies are in the pantry – so they down a bag of them. I always ask them the same question. Why are there cookies in the pantry in the first place? This brings me to a very important concept. Good choices start at the grocery store. So, when I am at the grocery store, I purchase food that is good for me and don't purchase crap. I look at the labels of what I buy and try to eat as much organic, raw and unprocessed foods as I can. If I can't find organic then I at least reach for natural products with no artificial ingredients and grass-fed, free-range or wild-caught lean animal proteins that are not loaded with antibiotics and hormones.

Do you know why lower quality animal products contain antibiotics? It's because the way they treat the animals. Mass production farms cram animals in small cages and the animals naturally get sick. You would too if you were treated this way. The stressful and unhealthy life these animals are forced to live takes a toll on their immune systems and they are susceptible to a variety of diseases. Because of this big corporations hit them up with antibiotics and steroids to keep them from dying and making them as big and meaty as possible. Not only does the animal live a horrible life but you get a crappy piece of meat or animal product (eggs, milk) that is filled with sickness and a variety of chemicals.

So, I always reach for free range, grass fed, steroid and antibiotic free or even better yet organic animal products. It may cost a little more but when it comes to my health I am willing to make that investment. Better to skimp on other things but not in this category.

To help offset the cost, I keep reminding myself how much I save not purchasing the sodas, alcohol, chips and candy and substituting good old filtered water and real food. Nature's secret weapon for aging well – H_2O! I also thought of how much I was saving from the reduced number of medical bills and time spent at the doctor. Several years ago, I was getting sick all the time. Once I started eating healthier I never got sick. That's real money saved and a much higher quality of life to boot!

I have more detailed information on good nutritional practices in *Chapter 6 – What you put in your stomach really does matter.*

Another note on basic health. I knew I had to do some form of exercise pretty much every day. I didn't have to be like our friend Arnold with massive biceps, that's pretty much a full time job, but I knew that I must move my body every day to be fit.

Don't always have time to exercise, I used to tell myself. I finally came to a point in my life that I just had to disagree with that statement. It all comes down to what I made a priority in my life. Little things I could do to increase my activity was to take the stairs and not the elevator or escalator. I don't search for the closest parking spot in front of the grocery store but park in the one furthest away. That always made me feel good as well since I was getting extra exercise and leaving that space next to the store or restaurant for someone who really could use it.

I also make sure I engage in a basic workout (30 – 60 minutes) six to seven days a week. I make sure I include cardio and resistance training. I personally like to run outside (I am an outside person) and weight-lift (but not as much as our friend Arnold does) and a quick yoga session at the end to stretch everything out.

I found mixing up the workouts really helped me and not to do the same thing over and over again. The body gets used to the routines and the mind gets very bored of it. Changing the workouts up really helps. Basically you can't make changes to your body working out on the elliptical three times a week at thirty minutes a pop. Not only are you going to be bored out of your mind but you aren't going to become healthier doing that.

So, not to tire you too much but eating healthier and working out has gone a long way to keeping me as young looking and feeling as possible. I'm not overdoing it or training like an Olympic athlete, but, basically, I need to have a plan that I can stick to for not just one week but for my whole life. More information on good ways to work out are included in *Chapter 5 – Keeping fit and working out.*

Also, the mind must be right to maximize results. I had to believe that I could accomplish my goals and then I could do the work to go after them. It's almost impossible to accomplish a goal without first having the dream to achieve that goal and the belief in that dream. I had to honestly believe that I could change so I did. It helps to keep a very positive attitude. Negativity goes a long way in stopping us from achieving our goals. So, the moral of the story is to stay positive and ignore the negativity. I give this my best shot every day.

That meant more potential changes were needed in my life. I had some negative *can't do* people in my circle and I had to remove myself from that toxic environment. I also had to remove people in my life that tried their very best to bring me down. There was no room for them in my life. Removing these negative people opened the door to find new positive people to be with. That was a big change in my life for the better – much more enjoyable. I just didn't need people in my life that brought me down and crush my dreams. So, I had to seek out those that encouraged my dreams and stay away from the nay-sayers. Believe me it helped me be the person I wanted to be. I mean if my so-called friends didn't encourage me in my quest to achieve my dreams were they really friends? If they talked about me behind my back in a negative way could I ever really trust them?

There is a quote in *The Bible* that mentions that if your hand is keeping you from being a good person then cut it off. *Matthew 5:0* in the *New Testament "and if thy right hand offend thee, cut it off, and cast it from thee."* I finally know what Matthew meant by that when I eliminated the negative people in my life. Just substitute *hand* with *negative people*. The result can be amazing.

Anyway, more on how the mind needs to be right is included in *Chapter 7 – The body cannot live without the mind.*

To close out this chapter (I told you I wouldn't bore you with a lot of words) I just want to mention that if you do follow any of the recommendations in this book, I warn you to not go overboard on any of these techniques. In doing so you run the risk of not being able to keep it up and giving up. Work up slowly, stay with the programs, be patient and you will get to where you want to be. Also, don't try to do everything at once. If you go from nothing to everything in one day you will find you won't have the time to do it all. Pick a few and get those done. Then move on to others.

I found that this is not a day-long journey but a life-time journey. I don't worry about being perfect and I learned not to beat myself up if I miss a day or two, and most importantly, I have fun with it.

I learned that I couldn't always push myself to be better every time I attempted something. For example, if I ran three miles today it didn't mean I should run four miles tomorrow and five the next day. The same holds true with weightlifting. I couldn't expect to up the weights every day. Otherwise I would be lifting far more than our friend, Arnold, and that's just not going to happen.

I had to learn the hard way, that if I did want to get better, then I did have to increase my weight, or activity, at times but I couldn't PR (personal record) every time I worked out. That mentality will only lead to disappointment and injury. It's about being smart and not getting hurt and letting the ego not get in the way. Better to take it slow and have the attitude to look forward to your activity and not to do it just to get it over with. Life is a journey and I knew that I had to enjoy that journey or I wasn't going to succeed.

This book is just a starting point so feel free to explore the areas I mention and other areas in more depth to find out what works for you. What works for me may not be the best solution for you. Invest some time in your greatest asset – *YOU!* If you do you will be more successful than Juan Ponce de León in his search for the Fountain of Youth.

Because you will actually find it.

Chapter 3 – Yes, you can really grow back your hair!

Pretty bold statement the title of this chapter is! And I can show you how I did it completely natural, so you can throw the Minoxidil (Rogaine) and Finasteride (Propecia) away! That last statement certainly won't be popular with the big drug companies but keeping them happy is not in my vision right now.

Being as healthy and clean and free of chemicals and poisons as I can possibly be is in my vision!

I also want to reiterate that this is about my journey through the Internet to find the secrets to looking and feeling years younger so I won't go into too much of the science behind why the techniques I share with you will restore your hair but I will touch on them and also point you in the right direction to where the real brains are behind this miracle cure of baldness.

I must say now that I am not an expert in this field, but as I mentioned above, I will let you know who they are. I wish I had their brain power but these individuals have done a lot of research and really know their stuff. They put in all the hours and we get to benefit from their work. I would listen to them.

I did.

I do need to caution you that it does take work and time. You probably won't see results for about five to six months and a real restoration in about ten months to a year or longer depending on where you are at when you start. So, if you have a small bald spot on the back of your head you should see full restoration before someone who is starting off completely bald (I was almost bald when I started). So just stay calm, do the work, have patience, enjoy the journey and you will get there. Trust me, you will.

So, I first started down this path when I saw an advertisement for a hair restoration e-book on the Internet about how to get my hair back naturally, without chemicals. The author was James Davis. I was intrigued but also skeptical, so I did a web search on reviews of this e-book. The reviews were decent, so I plunked down the money to read the book. The techniques didn't work perfectly for me but what works for you may not work for me and visa-versa, but the science behind why some of us go bald and some don't was very revealing.

I decided to do more investigating through the Internet and came to this web blogger: JD Moyer and his article on how he grew his hair back. The blog can be found here: *How I Thickened My Hair and Advanced My Hairline with a Simple Massage Technique (and no Drugs) at:* http://www.jdmoyer.com/2015/04/13/hair/.

Without taking too much of your time going over all the science, I will lay out some facts worth noting. First of all, we need to have some idea how baldness is caused before we can cure it. And the good news is there is a reason. JD Moyer mentions a paper he read from a different e-

22

book then the one I mentioned above. This e-book is from Rob (I don't know his last name) at www.perfecthairhealth.com. I subscribed to his free email course and eventually I bought his book. I must say the book was fascinating – more than just hair health but an overall approach to health.

JD Moyer and Rob mention a paper written by a coroner from Hong Kong. That paper can be found here: *Journal of Clinical & Experimental Dermatology Research: Detumescence Therapy of Human Scalp for Natural Hair Regrowth* at: https://www.omicsonline.org/detumescence-therapy-of-human-scalp-for-natural-hair-regrowth-2155-9554.1000138.pdf

This paper outlines the root cause of baldness and was written by Henry Choy. Choy, who studied the skulls of many deceased individuals, noticed that men who were bald had a thickening crud (yes that is not the scientific term) on their scalps. This crud is like cement that sits on top of the scalp. It's made of calcium and excess sebum (scalp oil). Men with full heads of hair did not have this crud.

So, what does hair need to have to be healthy? It needs oxygen and nutrients. How does it get oxygen and nutrients? From the blood supply. Now imagine a beautiful green lawn. The grass looks strong, thick, green and healthy. Now what do you think would happen if you poured a thin layer of cement over the grass? It would probably thin out some of the grass, right? Some may also turn brownish but still thrive. But not all of it would go away. Now what would happen if you added another layer of cement on top of the first layer? You would see less grass and browner grass. Not a healthy, thick, green carpet like it was before you added the cement. If the pattern continues then the grass would completely disappear (does this sound like male pattern baldness and premature graying of the hair)?

Why is this relevant? I think I just said it. Because this same idea is what's happening when someone goes bald (by the way Choy's study included women as well).

Now the big question is, yes, I have this calcification and sebum sludge in my scalp that's cutting off the blood supply to my hair basically killing it, what do I do now? How do I get rid of it so my hair can grow back?

Good question!

And there is an answer to that question as well!

Just cut your scalp open, scrape off the crud with a file, and then put your scalp back in place. Anyone can do this safely at home.
If you believe that you need to read *Chapter 7 – The body cannot live without the mind*. Because your mind is not right!

The real solution is a lot easier than that!

So, before we get into the solution, I have to state that eating a healthy diet is very helpful in growing hair and I suggest you eventually read *Chapter 6 – What you put in your stomach really does matter*, to get great tips on what to eat to promote hair growth as well as overall health. If you want more, Rob's book goes into more detail on the diet as well, so you can always purchase his book and read it yourself. Basically, there is a process to rid the calcium and excess sebum, but it won't do you any good if the blood going to your scalp and hair isn't carrying the proper nutrients.

Other than changing my diet to get the proper nutrients in the blood to feed the hair, how else can I help hair growth? The first thing you must do is get rid of the calcium and sebum blocking nutrient rich blood flow to your hair. So, I really don't suggest removing your scalp and I don't suggest going to a doctor to remove your scalp either. I don't think a doctor would actually do that anyway – probably lose their medical license if they did.

So, what can you do that's safe and right at home while you are watching TV? Here it is: You can perform two twenty minute scalp massages a day. One in the morning and one at night. How does this help? This will move the calcium and sebum sludge around, break it up, dissolve it and get it back to where it belongs – in the bone.

I'm not going to go into too much science here because you can get that from Rob (www.perfecthairhealth.com) or from JD Moyer at: *How I Thickened My Hair and Advanced My Hairline with a Simple Massage Technique (and no Drugs) at:* (http://www.jdmoyer.com/2015/04/13/hair/) but I will say this: Why is it that we lose our hair on top of our heads first and not on the sides or the face or the body? It's because we move those side and facial muscles around daily. Think about it. You smile, chew, walk, use your arms. You are moving that calcium sludge around and you are naturally dissolving it. But what about the top of your head? Not much movement going on so you must create the movement. There is also very little muscle to no muscle up on top of your scalp so working out the top of your head is nearly impossible.

Getting back to the massages. They also must be rough. This is not a feel good I'm going to get a head massage at the spa kind of massage. It's twenty minutes of beating up your scalp. This is the only way that it works. You need to crush up and dissolve the calcium and sebum in your scalp to get rid of it. The massage should include a vigorous warm up and just heating up the scalp and promoting blood flow. Then you need to pinch, press and stretch the skin on the scalp. It will be a bit painful, but you must do it to get blood flow to the hair.

So, start with basically massaging your hair and make sure you massage the whole scalp, not just the part where you have hair loss. Just warm up your scalp. After a few minutes start pinching your scalp. You can do this with one hand but I would suggest pinching with two hands. Basically, pushing the skin on the scalp together with a hand (fingers extended) on either side of the area (about ¼ to ½ inch apart). You want to try to actually lift the scalp skin off of your scalp. Do this all around your scalp for a few moments (about twice as long as your warm-up).

Once you are done with that you will press your scalp with your knuckles all around your scalp for about the same time (I actually now use an inexpensive hand held marble massage roller I got from my local running store by *Addaday:* www.addaday.com, to give my knuckles a break). Finally, you will stretch the skin on the scalp. Fundamentally, you are doing the opposite of the pinch method. Instead of pushing the skin together, you are pulling it away from each other. Do this all over your scalp as well. I then like to finish with a few more pinches and overall massaging the scalp.

For examples of these techniques check our *Rob's Perfect Hair Health* site at www.Perfecthairhealth.com and sign up for Rob's email course. You will be glad you did.

Now I must admit that for me the massage in the morning is harder to complete time-wise because it gets in the way of getting all the other things I need to get done in the morning before going to work (eating breakfast, showering, working out, etc.) but getting my hair back was important enough to me so I found a way most of the time to get it in. I have to admit, however, sometimes the morning massage only lasted around six to ten minutes.

The evening massage is easier. I usually do it after dinner when I'm watching TV. And the way the people in this country watch TV it should be easy to slip in 20 minutes.

So, with all this said your hair will, more than likely, get worse in the first few months. Mine did. I think mine appeared to get worse because I quickly lost the weaker (and dying) hairs that were barely hanging on from the rigorous massage. But I was willing to sacrifice that short-term backwards slide to achieve long-term gain of healthy hair.

Most people, including myself, experienced dandruff and oily hair when performing these massages in the beginning. This is completely normal, and the oily hair usually means you are actually squeezing out some of the excess sebum through the scalp. This is a good thing.

Now along with this you shouldn't wash your hair every day. I moved to once per week from my once or twice daily. At first this seemed weird and my hair felt a little oily but then the hair and scalp adjusted and I found I could keep my hair clean by mainly washing it with water alone. Rob at *Perfect Hair Health:* www.perfecthairhealth.com actually recommends not using shampoo or conditioner ever and just using water but I haven't gone total "hippie" yet. That's probably why Rob's mane looks a lot better than mine.

I do use natural and organic shampoos, however, with no sulfites that can damage the hair. I think reducing the amount of times I shampoo, along with the organic shampoo, has helped tremendously. I get this shampoo from a health food store. In my case I get it at Whole Foods but I'm sure most organic markets will sell organic shampoo and conditioner or you can get it on the Internet.

When you start the massages, you will also likely notice that your scalp skin is very tight. This is due to the calcium buildup on the skull that pulls the skin on the scalp tight (think of plastic wrap loosely over a container but then you keep putting stuff into the container and the plastic wrap stretches and gets tighter and tighter). Therefore, most bald men have domed shaped scalps and the skin becomes tight. If you are consistent with the scalp massaging you will notice that the skin on your scalp will start to loosen. Don't worry this is a good thing! It means you are breaking up and dissolving the calcium under the scalp and the skin is not being pulled tight by the excess calcium.

Around month five you should start to see some new hair growth, but I need to let you know that new hair growth comes in very thin at first and is basically white. As it matures the hair shaft will darken to your hair color and thicken. Also, new hair grows very slowly. Think of how hair grows on a newborn baby. It's thin and frail at first but then thickens and darkens over time. Therefore, the process of *re-growing* hair takes a while. You will notice the new hair doesn't grow as fast as the other hair you already have. Don't worry, after a while it will grow the same.

If you have average hair loss then around month ten you should see about eighty percent of your hair return. If you were completely bald when you started it will take significantly longer. The good news is, if you keep up the massages, there's no reason you shouldn't be able to get it all back. It can be as soon as a year or as long as three depending on where you were when you started. But it's never too late to start. I'm living proof of that! Here are some photos starting on the next page of my progress:

Day 1

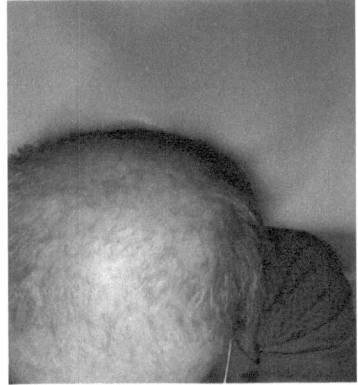

8 Months

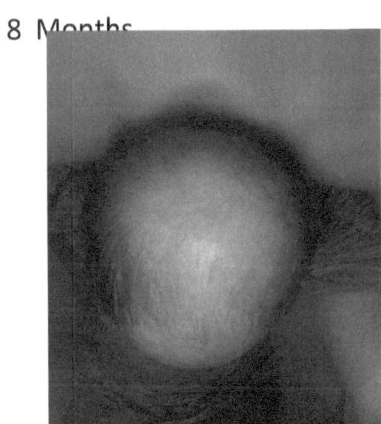

1 year

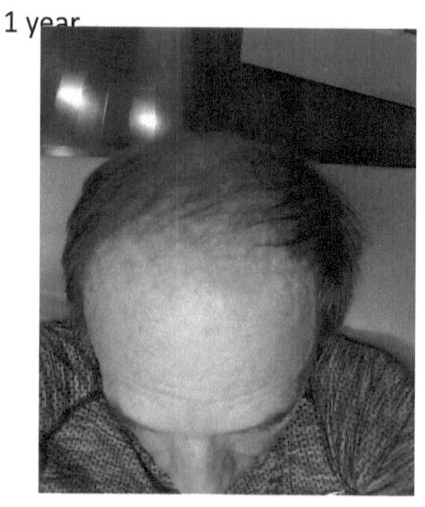

1 ½ Year

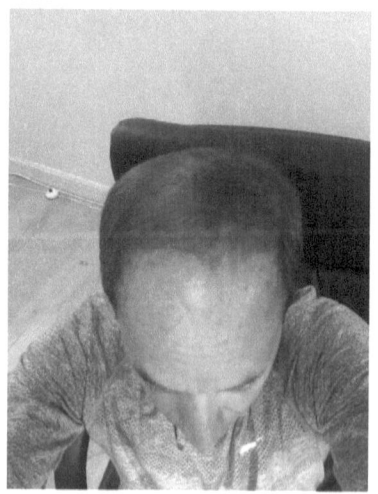

So, to summarize, you need to perform two twenty-minute massages consistently every day (morning and evening). You need to really massage the scalp by rubbing, pinching, pressing (I use my knuckles or a massage roller) and stretching the skin. You need to give it at least ten months to see the best results. You should also be eating well – see *Chapter 6 – What you put in your stomach really does matter*, for more information on nutrition or refer to Rob's book and website at *Perfect Hair Health* (www.perfecthairhealth.com).

If you want to see a video of how to do the massage techniques, or would like more information on this topic, I would suggest purchasing Rob's book at *Perfect Hair Health at* www.perfecthairhealth.com. No, I don't get a commission on this book and I don't even know Rob personally (I don't even know his last name)! I just got a lot out of his book and it worked for me and the cost of the book is a lot less than a prescription of Minoxidil.

But I gave you enough to grow your hair back so you should be good if you follow these procedures.

Moving on, since our bodies are made up of a lot of water, I recommend that you drink a lot of water. How much you ask? Most people would say 8 eight-ounce glasses a day (total of 8 x 8 = 64 ounces per day).

I never liked that answer.

I just can't believe the water need is the same for a 90-pound female gymnast as it is for a 250-pound male body builder. It obviously depends on your weight and activity level. As a rule of thumb, I like to take my weight and multiply by 2/3 to come up with the total ounces to drink per day. For me it would be 150 lbs. x 2/3 = 100 ounces a day. The average bottle of water has about sixteen ounces in it so a little more than six of those bottles a day would be right for me. I also will add an additional twelve ounces for every thirty minutes of working out on top of that. I learned these tidbits from the article that can be found here from Slender Kitchen: *How to Calculate How Much Water You Should Drink A Day,* by <u>Kristen Mccaffrey</u> at: <u>http://www.slenderkitchen.com/article/how-to-calculate-how-much-water-you-should-drink-a-day</u>.

There are other sites on the Internet that will recommend anywhere from ½ ounce to 1 full ounce of water per day per body weight. I would experiment to see what works well for you. The 2/3 version works for me. I would start there and then modify for what works for you.

To make it easier, I have water bottles everywhere. One on a table next to my bed, one in my basement where I work out, one in my office next to my computer, one in both of my cars and one on the table in the family room where I watch television. That's seven bottles of water spread out around my house and cars! I always use filtered water so I'm not getting all the impurities from tap water and filtered water just tastes better. I also carry around a large Hydro Flask® (basically a big metal can) almost everywhere I go so I have no excuse not to get the water in. The other seven bottles are actually just for back up in case I don't have my Hydro Flask® with me. Which does happen more often than it should.

You don't have to be this fanatical about the water but just make sure you get your recommended amount in every day.

Just be prepared to pee a lot – I mean A LOT! And I know this may be gross but a good indicator to see if you are well enough hydrated is to inspect your pee. If it's clear like water with a very slight yellow hue you are doing great. If it's dark yellow, then drink some water and if it's brown stop everything and drink a lot of water! If it's completely clear (not likely) like water with absolutely no yellow hue you are probably overdoing the drinking a bit. A great chart can be found in this article from the Cleveland Clinic: *What The Color of Your Urine Says About You: Color, density, and smell can reveal health problems* at: https://health.clevelandclinic.org/2013/10/what-the-color-of-your-urine-says-about-you-infographic/.

I can't leave this chapter without also talking about hair masks and oils that make some outlandish claims on how you can grow inches of hair everyday if you use the mask or oil. Don't expect miracles to happen overnight! There is so much information on the Internet regarding this topic it's absolutely mind blowing. Don't believe me? Go to *Youtube* at www.youtube.com and search on DIY masks for hair growth. DIY, I found out later, means: *do it yourself*.

Now I don't know Rob from *Perfect Hair Health* at www.perfecthairhealth.com personally but, after reading his book, I believe he would simply roll his eyes if I said this in his presence, but I would look into some of these. You can see some masks that come up more than others (more popular with youtubers) or different masks that share common ingredients and you can see reviews from those who tried the remedies and see what their experiences with the masks were. One I do like is Annie Jaffery's use of coconut oil for a head massage as well as a moisturizer. You can find her youtube video at: *DIY Scalp Massage for Healthy Strong Hair!* ♥ *(Stimulates Growth & Conditions)* at https://www.youtube.com/watch?v=C9LpfBEkF7s. Annie also has other great tips on general health, fitness & wellness and you can find her channel at: https://www.youtube.com/user/AnnieJaffrey.

I'm going to list a few others below in my section of other steps you can take if the massages aren't 100% working for you. We are all different and our bodies react differently so not everything is going to work the same for everyone.

Also, after viewing a few of these videos on hair masks you may make up some of your own. I like to take a mixture of coconut oil, lemon juice, castor oil and olive oil and top it off with a few drops of peppermint oil and frankincense oil. I massage that in my scalp. I've been doing the mask for a while now and I do believe I see a benefit in overall hair health. Anyway, if you are interested you can do your own searches and I know you will find all sorts of variations. Just remember that if you do this, you should use organic and nature food products (my coconut oil is actually organic and unrefined). If you do I don't think you can hurt yourself. These ingredients are just clean food items.

I will put the oil on my hair and actually sleep with it on almost every night (although I do take breaks from this habit, especially if I'm traveling). That way I get all the nutritional benefits all night long. If you want to try this but don't want to have it on your scalp and hair all night long, I would suggest leaving it on for at least an hour before washing the mask out.

To find out what works for you will take experimentation so have fun with it and give any of these at least a few months to see if they are working. Just keep your expectations realistic. As I mentioned before, there are some Youtube videos that will claim phenomenal results overnight. Any claim that states you will see a difference in one night is crazy. At least that was and continues to be my observation. Just have patience.

Remember you have to sow, cultivate and then harvest. So many of us want instant gratification and skip the cultivate part but that is a very important part of the process. Life is a journey, not an end-point and it takes going through the journey to get where you want to be. Who knows, you may even surpass your original goals and go for more!

Even our good friend Arnold had to go through a lot of work to transform his body, it didn't come in one night, so I knew when I started on my journey to regrow my hair that it wasn't going to happen overnight.

Now, with all that said, as my hair started to come back, I became a little restless. A bit contradictory to what I just stated but I really wanted my hair to grow back faster – who wouldn't? So I kept researching the web to see if there were any other ideas out there that can help with hair growth and I will cover those now.

Dermarolling:

So I never heard of dermarolling before I started my journey to grow my hair back but a dermaroller is a device with many (around 190) microneedles that creates micro pinpricks in the scalp or skin. They come with different needle sizes (0.1mm to 2.0mm). You can actually use dermarollers on your scalp for hair growth or on your face, neck and hands for collagen growth. The way this works is that it temporarily injures your scalp or skin, tricking the body to send more blood and nutrients to that area to *heal* it. In doing so, the blood brings more nutrients to your hair as well, tricking the hair to grow.

Typically you use a longer needle for the scalp (0.5mm to 1.5mm) than on the face and hands (0.2mm to 0.5mm).

A photo of the dermaroller is here:

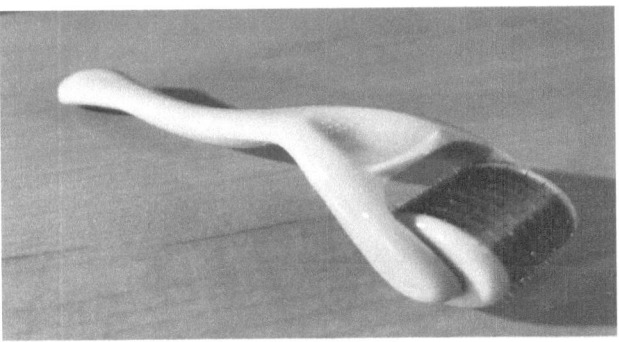

This specific dermaroller has 192 microneedles with a length of 1mm. This is the one that I started with on my scalp. I eventually graduated to a 1.5mm dermaroller with the same amount of microneedles.

To use the dermaroller you need to roll this device on your scalp. Make sure to clean your scalp very well and clean and sterilize the dermaroller with rubbing alcohol. This is a very important step because if you don't you can run into infection!

But don't worry, if you do it right, dermarolling is a safe, effective way to help regrow your hair and to make it healthier.

Dermarolling worked better for me when I wet my hair to keep it down while rolling my scalp. That way the hair doesn't get in the way or get tangled and break during the dermaroller process.

I go over the entire scalp in 4 different directions. I first go front to back, lifting the dermaroller and starting again from the front (some people go back and forth but I don't want to take a chance of breaking the hair shaft). I do this from one side to the other to cover the entire scalp (front, top, back and sides).

Next I roll at a 90 degree angle from the first set of rolls (basically side to side). Again I do this to cover the entire scalp. Then I roll diagonal one way then diagonal the other way, covering the scalp completely, not just the bald spots.

Now I have to say that this hurts a little (a lot at first but then you get used to it). At least that was my experience. Others with a higher pain tolerance may not feel it at all. Most of us, however, will feel something.

Think about it, you are punching hundreds of small holes in your scalp! Some people use a numbing cream but I never did. As I mentioned, dermarolling actually gets easier over time. If you do use a numbing cream remember to wipe the numbing cream off of your scalp before you start dermarolling. You don't want the numbing cream to enter into the holes in scalp that the dermaroller makes.

You should see your scalp or skin that you are dermarolling become red. This is perfectly normal and is due to increased blood flow to the area. This is a good thing. You may also see a small amount of blood, but don't worry about that, it won't hurt you in the long run and it just shows that blood is coming up to your scalp and *feeding* your hair!

If you use the 1mm needle dermaroller I would do this once every two weeks. If you use the 1.5mm needle dermaroller I would do once every three weeks. There are many different opinions out there on the Internet so you need to review and experiment with these and see which process works best for you. The good things is, there are several good Youtube (www.youtube.com) videos on dermarolling out there in Youtube land.

I watched a few videos but the one I thought was the most insightful was from Reborn Hair PPP (https://www.youtube.com/channel/UCVRBe1B_2JzvB_4Y-c1qvUw/featured?disable_polymer=1) at *How to Regrow Your Hair With A Dermaroller Properly* at: https://www.youtube.com/watch?v=yaKhKlyavA4. This video also gets deep into the science of the effects of the dermaroller so I recommend watching this video before trying the dermarolling process.

Another good video to view for spot dermarolling (not the whole scalp but just the areas that are thinning) can be found on Sheetal's youtube channel: (https://www.youtube.com/user/purplefish3/featured?disable_polymer=1) at *HOW TO REGROW HAIR WITH A DERMA ROLLER│DERMA ROLLING SCALP FOR FASTER HAIR GROWTH │GROW THIN HAIR!* at: https://www.youtube.com/watch?v=ynSDiDz-Sbo. She is also very positive and that's a good thing. We need more of that in the world!

Inversion Method:

The inversion method seems to be getting some real play in the hair growth guru's venue out there in hair growth guru land. The science makes sense. What you do is warm up some oil (I usually use coconut or grapeseed oil for this or some other elaborate concoction I'll discuss below) and massage it gently (not like the aggressive massages mentioned earlier) into your scalp. While doing this you are going to sit forward in a chair, bent at the waist, with your head between your legs as low to the floor as you can handle. You can also do a headstand or have your legs on a sofa and have the top portion of your body tilt towards the floor and prop up with elbows (sort of like sphinx position but your legs are on a coach and your elbows are on the floor. The important thing is to have your head below your heart. Also make sure the oil is warm but not hot. You don't want to burn yourself.

When having your head below your heart, your blood will flow faster to your scalp and therefore deliver more oxygen and nutrients to your scalp, feeding your hair. The recommended amount of time is four minutes.

I wouldn't try this if you have any medical issues without first checking with your doctor. If you are in fine health, with no blood pressure issues, then you should be fine, but again, if you have any doubts please check with your doctor. Common sense prevails here so if you find yourself getting dizzy or nauseated when upside down then this might not be the best method for you.

Below is picture of me displaying the inversion method:

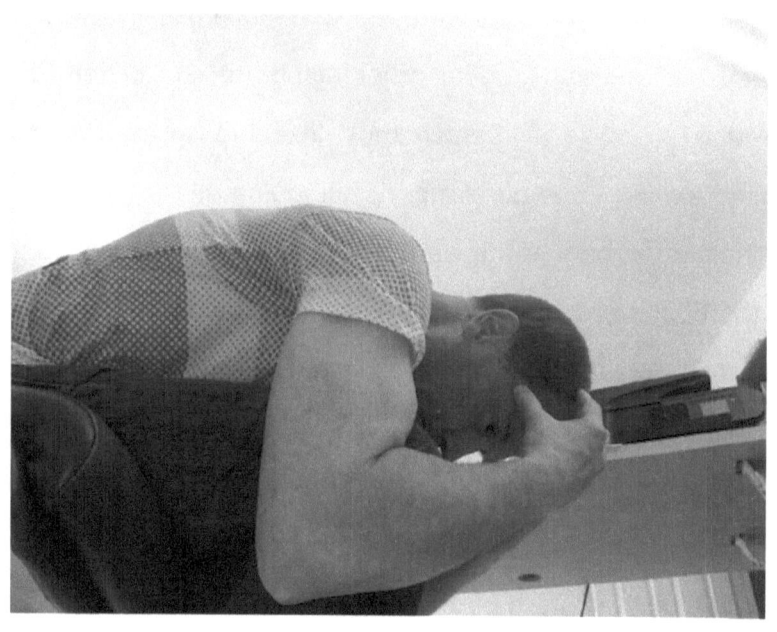

There is a very good youtube video: *The Science of the Inversion Method | NATURAL HAIR* (https://www.youtube.com/watch?v=PjqmZkiyL6o) by Green Beauty at: (https://www.youtube.com/channel/UCsjtadigSejJvFJOQh1myMw). Take a look and feel free to research other videos on this topic.

Another good video on a hair oil can be found on EricTipsReviews! (https://www.youtube.com/channel/UCEP2Salwz1kLMp292iOfW_w) at: *Grow THICKER HAIR NATURALLY with oils!!!!* (https://www.youtube.com/watch?v=1v2PRuxoMp8). Eric's recipe incorporates six different oils and each oil brings something to facilitate hair growth. I've made this recipe and I have to say I'm very happy with it. The oils he uses are: coconut, Emu, jojoba, sweet almond, caster & vitamin E. I've also made this recipe but replaced the Emu oil with olive oil. Partly because I like the benefits olive oil brings to the table and I feel a little bad for the Emus that give up their lives just for the oil. I also put in a few drops of peppermint oil and frankincense oil. I would definitely recommend you giving this concoction or the many others in youtube (www.youtube.com) a try!

So, in summary, there are many methods to get your hair back. From my experience, Rob's Perfect Hair Health (www.Perfecthairhealth.com) is the most solid way to go and his book has the most amount of research and science behind it. I would definitely go that route and add in some of the other methods mentioned in this book to assist with his program.

I got my hair back, if you follow these methods there is a good chance you will also.

Chapter 4 - Wrinkles – don't worry we will get rid of them

So, when I was researching my hair problem on the Internet, I noticed that all sorts of other *recommended* searches popped up. I initially dismissed these but then reminded myself that I should have an open mind and it wouldn't hurt to, at the very least, investigate the possibilities of some of these recommendations.

Some of these recommendations had to do with *anti-aging* (or my preferred phrase, *aging-well*) and the elimination of wrinkles on the face, neck and hands. As I mentioned earlier, I noticed that I was aging faster than I thought I should be and I decided to go down the rabbit hole through the Internet to find some potential remedies to assist me in my plight to stave off the negative effects of aging.

Now don't get me wrong, I don't mind getting older (considering the alternative) but I, and I'm sure I'm not alone, don't like everything that comes with age. Maybe you are okay with it, but I'd rather fix this issue and become the best version of myself as possible. So, I rolled up my sleeves and diligently went to work on discovering some possible solutions.

After a good amount of research I came up with a little theory on why some of us see the negative parts of aging over others and what can be done to help slow down the negative effects of aging. But before I divulge that notion I have to ask a question. Why is it that our faces get wrinkly and old well before our rumps do? I think most of us know one of the reasons, but I think there is at least one other reason and with a few lifestyle changes I believe we can slow down and reverse what has been done over the years.

So, what are my two theories that are the result of aging prematurely? Number one theory we should all know. As much as I like the sun (and I think it's important to soak it up for the vitamin D3 effect) I try very hard not to have too much of it on my face, neck or hands. Because of this, I limit the sun as much as possible on those specific areas. You see, those areas are the most exposed areas on the body, they typically will get enough sunlight no matter what you do, unless you live in a cave. But make sure you get a good amount of our friend, the sun, on other areas of your bodies (I know this is controversial but I believe it's true). For more about the sun please see *Chapter 8 – The sun is not all that bad for you (did I just say that)?* So, moving on ...

I use a good sunscreen that protects against UVA & UVB rays. I usually look for a natural version at a heath store or Whole Foods and around SPF 30 or higher. I don't like smearing chemicals all over my body so I stay away from the big named brands. I also wear a good pair of sunglasses (the cheap ones do nothing to protect you) and sometimes a hat – especially in my bald days but now that my hair has grown back not so much.

Now for the little known other cause for wrinkles. The face actually has muscle under it. But unlike the muscles in the rest of our body they are not used as much. I mean how much do you use your forehead muscles? So, in order to reduce the number of wrinkles on your face, chin and neck you need to work out and massage those areas just like you would work out your arms, shoulders, chest, back and legs.

And if you are not working out your other body muscles you need to read *Chapter – 5 Keeping fit and working out* – just saying.

As I mentioned before, I am no expert in anything. Just ask my wife and son they can attest to this. They would actually be happy to! But this book is about my journey through the Internet to find the fountain of youth, not a debate on my intelligence. Here is what I found during my search.

There is a lot of great material on the World Wide Web to show you facial massages and exercises that will help you reduce and eliminate wrinkles and it's all just sitting on the Internet for you to review and use for free. I'm going to share with you the ones I felt helped me the most. I would suggest starting with these and then branching out if you want to.

I first started with Patricia Goroway's *Facial Fitness* (https://www.facialfitnesssystem.com). You can find a great video here: *Facial Fitness System by Patricia Goroway_____at:*

What I like about this version of Patricia's video is that she educates the viewer regarding the muscles of the face. Then she demonstrates her exercises and lets you know what muscles are working and how to perform the exercises. After showing the basic exercises she then goes over some more advanced facial exercises before finishing up with facial massage techniques.

I think starting with her video is a great way to begin your journey to reduce and eliminate wrinkles. You can also review Patricia's site *FACIAL FITNESS SYSTEM* at http://www.facialfitnesssystem.com/ for more on the topic.

After working with Patricia's videos for a month or so, I then branched out and reviewed several other sites before finding a couple more I really like. There is a site by a woman who used to call herself the Vitalitist (Now Xuan Barbara) that has a great routine. You can get to her Youtube channel here: https://www.youtube.com/channel/UCzSyRtVwCdtXwyFYMy6sQrA.

I really like her video: *Facial Yoga – Full lesson 2* at: https://www.youtube.com/watch?v=Nsxr4OTc0kA. This is a great video that is packed with a bunch of different facial exercises and believe me you will feel the burn! It's a great compliment to Patricia's video because they work on slightly different parts of the face. In my humble opinion, Patricia seems to focus on the neck and jaw, although she does a great job with the whole face, and Xuan Barbara's is a little more rigorous on the whole face. In fact, my face is actually exhausted after performing her routine.

I'll go over my schedule with these videos after I share one more website with you. So far, we have mainly discussed facial exercises (or facial yoga). Although Patricia has a massage portion and Xuan Barbara incorporates some massages in her routine, there is another great series of videos I came across that focuses solely on facial massage. There is a young lady who I believe, name is Olga Toja, has a great Youtube channel at: *Olgatoja:* https://www.youtube.com/user/olgatoja. She has some great videos on facial massage. She has other healthy lifestyle videos up on her page as well.

Now that I shared that with you I'll go over my daily schedule (when I first started out) shown on the next page.

Facial Exercise & Massage Schedule

Day	Time of day	Video Title	Type	Duration (min)	Instructor	Website
1	Morning	Forehead Wrinkles Massage - Do It While You Watch It	Massage	5.21	Olgatoja	https://www.youtube.com/watch?v=R1NoMDJAYLQ
1	Morning	Eye Wrinkles Massage - Do It While You Watch It	Massage	4.45	Olgatoja	https://www.youtube.com/watch?v=YfQ7cp2vkpI
1	Morning	Smile Wrinkles Massage - Do It While You Watch It	Massage	7.09	Olgatoja	https://www.youtube.com/watch?v=EBs4uhEBdf8
1	Morning	How to Get Rid Of Double Chin Fast With Face Massage | Neck Fat Reduction Without Surgery	Massage	8.00	Olgatoja	https://www.youtube.com/watch?v=NQo3gELng-k
1	Morning	Facial Fitness	Exercises	25.06	Patricia Goroway	https://www.youtube.com/watch?v=0diJ1hx4lbI&list=PLnvpR2oTa8rlMLf5cZ5lvHQ0cEr3AiLbE
1	Evening	Forehead Wrinkles Massage - Do It While You Watch It	Massage	5.21	Olgatoja	https://www.youtube.com/watch?v=R1NoMDJAYLQ
1	Evening	Eye Wrinkles Massage - Do It While You Watch It	Massage	4.45	Olgatoja	https://www.youtube.com/watch?v=YfQ7cp2vkpI
1	Evening	Smile Wrinkles Massage - Do It While You Watch It	Massage	7.09	Olgatoja	https://www.youtube.com/watch?v=EBs4uhEBdf8
1	Evening	How to Get Rid Of Double Chin Fast With Face Massage | Neck Fat Reduction Without Surgery	Massage	8.00	Olgatoja	https://www.youtube.com/watch?v=NQo3gELng-k
2	Morning	Forehead Wrinkles Massage - Do It While You Watch It	Massage	5.21	Olgatoja	https://www.youtube.com/watch?v=R1NoMDJAYLQ
2	Morning	Eye Wrinkles Massage - Do It While You Watch It	Massage	4.45	Olgatoja	https://www.youtube.com/watch?v=YfQ7cp2vkpI
2	Morning	Smile Wrinkles Massage - Do It While You Watch It	Massage	7.09	Olgatoja	https://www.youtube.com/watch?v=EBs4uhEBdf8
2	Morning	How to Get Rid Of Double Chin Fast With Face Massage | Neck Fat Reduction Without Surgery	Massage	8.00	Olgatoja	https://www.youtube.com/watch?v=NQo3gELng-k
2	Morning	Facial Yoga – Full lesson 2	Exercises	23.26	Xuan Barbara	https://www.youtube.com/watch?v=Nsxr4OTcOkA
2	Evening	Forehead Wrinkles Massage - Do It While You Watch It	Massage	5.21	Olgatoja	https://www.youtube.com/watch?v=R1NoMDJAYLQ
2	Evening	Eye Wrinkles Massage - Do It While You Watch It	Massage	4.45	Olgatoja	https://www.youtube.com/watch?v=YfQ7cp2vkpI
2	Evening	Smile Wrinkles Massage - Do It While You Watch It	Massage	7.09	Olgatoja	https://www.youtube.com/watch?v=EBs4uhEBdf8
2	Evening	How to Get Rid Of Double Chin Fast With Face Massage | Neck Fat Reduction Without Surgery	Massage	8.00	Olgatoja	https://www.youtube.com/watch?v=NQo3gELng-k

Now I realize this looks like a lot but once you perform them a couple of times you are going to skip through to the parts you need so it actually takes up less time then it shows here. Also notice the chart breaks out day 1 and day 2. I basically started with the massages twice a day and one of the exercise routines. I rotate the exercises between the two: Patricia Goroway's and Xuan Barbara's or a different routine.

So again, it may look like a lot but it really doesn't take up that much time. Especially since doing these routines should help to erase years on your face or at least slow the effects of aging. I believe it's worth it!

I sometimes substitute another video I found for the evening massage. There is a lady named Dr. Mona Vand (Youtube channel https://www.youtube.com/channel/UC0GkEyks1Nnzhsi9bCZTIjA) who has some great videos as well. Her facial massage video can be found here: *Anti-aging Face Lifting Massage | Dr Mona Vand* at https://www.youtube.com/watch?v=whCvshXaVe4.

I now only do the massage in the morning. I think once you have done the massages for a few months you can do less of them as you go from change mode to maintenance mode. I also only do the facial exercises about three times a week for the same reason mentioned above.

I would like to share two other facial exercise videos I came across when I was finishing up with this book. The video is from: *Glow Healthy with* *Chelsea* (https://www.youtube.com/channel/UCo2L4i5mLFXjnpe5JNQXz9Q)

called *Facial Yoga - Full Routine (Face Exercises and Massage)* at https://www.youtube.com/watch?v=GgXwSphZ9bE&t=51s and her update to that video: *Facial Yoga 2.0 - Full Routine (Anti Aging Face Exercises) Updated Workout* at https://www.youtube.com/watch?v=q9x7xamaBfM.

These are a good substitute to *Facial Yoga – Full lesson 2* mentioned above if you want to change it up a bit. Remember, change is good.

I also want to state that I didn't beat myself up if I missed a routine – I just don't worry about it. I knew that if I honestly tried to do this every day, but skipped a day here and there, that I was doing great. If I could only squeak out the massages in the morning and not in the evening as well it's ok. I was still doing better than the majority of the population which is doing, you guessed it, nothing!

I'm going to go over this a lot in the book. If you try to follow what I do, just try your best but don't beat yourself up if you don't get everything done in a day. Just make an honest attempt at it and do the best you can.

During my journey, I found myself shortening the routines based on how much time I had. Sometimes there is more than one exercise for a particular part of the face, so sometimes I would cut out an exercise here and there. I just made sure to do at least one exercise per face part. I also reduced the number of reps per exercise if I was in a hurry (aren't we all) and go through the whole routine. Then when I had more time I would go back to the full routine with the recommended reps.

In conclusion, if you want to follow what I have done, I would suggest you start with these videos and then venture out. There are new ones coming out every day. Just know that you have to be doing them consistently for about three months to start seeing real results and if you keep doing them you will keep seeing results. Unfortunately, when you stop doing these exercises and massages you will go back to where you were before. Therefore, make sure to pick a routine you believe you can live with your whole life. In other words, don't overdo it or you will surely quit. More is not always more if you know what I mean.

And just remember that these are the routines that work for me. You may find others on the Internet that work better for you and your lifestyle and that's perfectly fine. We are all different: women, men, young, middle-aged, elderly, heavy, light, tall, short, full-time job, unemployed, retired, student, athlete, etc. There is not one program that fits all, just like a piece of apparel. So, I did some customization to make these programs work for me personally.

I would also like to mention that there is a boatload of information out on www.youtube.com on DIY (do it yourself) facemasks. I've tried many of these and created my own. These include making a mask (I use all organic) from food products that you can use on your face, hands, neck, hair and all over your body. The idea is to bring moisture and nutrients to the skin to reduce wrinkles and promote healthy, glowing skin. Skin is our largest organ so we need to keep it healthy.

I don't substitute the massaging or facial exercising for the masks, however. I look at it as icing on the cake!

The majority of these DIY masks incorporate coconut oil. But some include other household ingredients. A few that I've come across are: turmeric (fresh is better than powder), avocado, raw honey, castor oil, olive oil, vitamin E (liquid form), fermented rice water, plain Greek yogurt, star anise, sweet almond oil, grapeseed oil, jojoba oil, rice water, aloe vera – the list goes on and on. If you want to follow me on any of these, I will put up some on www.youtube.com and I would suggest researching other Youtube videos. I would also read the comments and reviews associated with the videos. Some of these recipes receive more praise than others so I picked the ones with good reviews, so you may want to do the same. Have fun with it and experiment. Who knows, you may end up with your own concoction that works wonders.

For an example, here is a video from Dr. Mona Vand (https://www.youtube.com/channel/UC0GkEyks1Nnzhsi9bCZTIjA) with a Turmeric mask: *Turmeric DIY Beauty Mask | Dr Mona Vand:* https://www.youtube.com/watch?v=t1Qma-p91Cs.

Now, I've covered the face but what about the neck and hands? Along with the face these are the other body parts that appear old quicker than the rest of our body parts due to being exposed to the elements more than the other body parts.

I don't have much to say on this topic other than I typically will do for the neck and hands whatever I do for the face. Any mask I put on my face I also use it on my neck and hands. I noticed it's helped in curing damaged skin on these areas. I also use natural sunscreen for the neck and hands the same exact way I use it for my face. The sun can be a great friend and I love it (provides vitamin D) but you need to protect yourself and your face, neck and hands are in the sun more than any other body parts. For more on the benefits of sun exposure see *Chapter 8 – The sun is not all that bad for you (did I just say that)?*

Another item I use is a Clarisonic. You can find the info here: https://www.clarisonic.com/. This is a great exfoliating brush that I use every day on my face, neck and hands. I just add it to my morning shower routine and it only takes a couple of minutes. I really feel clean after using this device. There are some good tips on this Youtube video: *The Clarisonic Bible: 10 Things You Need to Know ASAP!* At: https://www.youtube.com/watch?v=uhgOla2i9cw&t=116s from a Youtuber called Popsugar Beauty (https://www.youtube.com/channel/UCN781-j50kA-q2CsGqZuzlg). This video outlines some good do's and don'ts when it comes to using the device.

Another crazy routine out there that I have tried and still do on occasion is dermarolling. I touch on dermarolling in *Chapter 3 – Yes, you can really grow back your hair!* But I found that people are definitely using the dermaroller on the face, neck and hands as well. Why? To build collagen and bring blood and nutrients to those areas. This helps in the reduction in wrinkles and imperfections in those areas.

See a pattern here?

But maybe you didn't read *Chapter 3 – Yes, you can really grow back your hair!* Because you have a full head of hair. So I will go over what the dermaroller is right now.

A dermaroller is a device with many (around 190) microneedles that creates micro pinpricks in the scalp or skin (depending on what you want out of it). Dermarollers come with different needle sizes. (0.1mm to 2.0mm). So you can actually use dermarollers on your scalp for hair growth or on your face, neck and hands for collagen growth. The way this works is that it temporarily injures your scalp or skin, tricking the body to send more blood and nutrients to that area to *heal* it and helping the body to eliminate wrinkles and imperfections in the skin.

Typically you use a longer needle for the scalp (0.5mm to 1.5mm) than on the face and hands (0.2mm to 1.5mm). I wouldn't start with anything longer than 0.5mm.

A photo of the dermaroller is here:

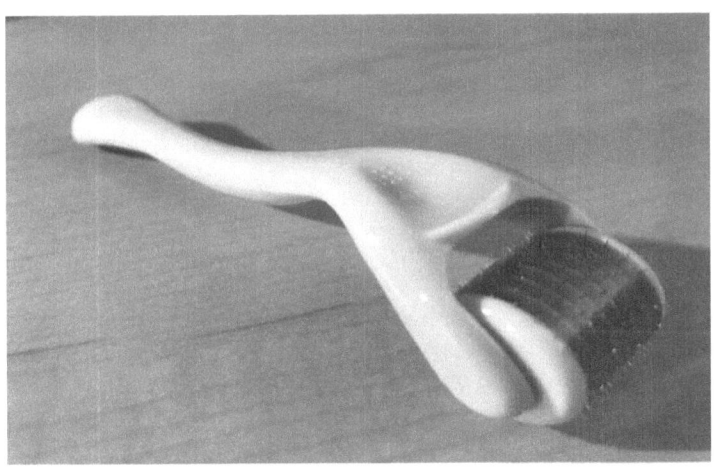

This specific dermaroller has 192 microneedles with a length of 0.5mm. This is the one that I use for my face, neck and hands.

To use the dermaroller you need to roll this device on your face, neck and hands. Make sure to clean those areas very well and clean and sterilize the dermaroller with rubbing alcohol. This is a very important step because if you don't you can run into infection!

But don't worry, if you do it right, dermarolling is a safe, effective way to help your skin become healthier, brighter and younger.

I go over the area (face, neck and hands) in 4 different directions. I first go front to back, in a back and forth movement. I do this from one side to the other to cover the entire area.

Next I roll at a 90 degree angle from the first set of rolls (basically side to side). Again I do this to cover the entire area. Then I roll diagonal one way then diagonal the other way, covering the area completely. I will do the face first, then the neck, then the hands.

Now I have to say that this hurts a little (a lot at first but then you get used to it). At least that was my experience. Others with a higher pain tolerance may not feel it at all. Most of us, however, will feel something!

Think about it, you are punching hundreds of small holes in your skin! Some people use a numbing cream but I never did. As I mentioned, dermarolling actually gets easier over time. If you do use a numbing cream remember to wipe it off before you start dermarolling. You don't want the numbing cream to enter into the holes in skin that the dermaroller makes. That's not a good idea.

You should see your skin that you are dermarolling become red. This is perfectly normal and is due to increased blood flow to the area.

This is a good thing. You may also see a small amount of blood, but don't worry about that, it won't hurt you in the long run and it just shows that blood is coming up to your face, neck or hands bringing nourishment to those areas!

If you use the 0.5mm needle dermaroller I would do this once every six weeks (you need time so the skin can heal). Some people actually do this as much as every two weeks. There are different opinions on the Internet so you need to review and experiment with these and see which process works best for you. The good thing is, there are several good Youtube (www.youtube.com) videos on dermarolling out there in Youtube land.

I watched a few videos but the one I thought was the most insightful was from *Beauty by Anne-Marie* (https://www.youtube.com/watch?v=6dOuPz7KNQs) at *Dermarolling FULL face, hands, neck and lips! DEMO* at: https://www.youtube.com/watch?v=6dOuPz7KNQs. This video also gets deep into the science of the effects of the dermaroller so I recommend watching this video before trying the dermarolling process.

Another good video to look at that shows that men can do this as well can be found on James Welch's youtube channel : (https://www.youtube.com/channel/UCPP291gN79qI1QZY1znOscg) at *Derma Rolling - Remove Acne Scars, Dark Spots, Fine Lines, Pigmentation (oily skin)* ✘ *James Welsh* at: https://www.youtube.com/watch?v=pjeHU4ZtObY&t=277s. He has other helpful videos on general skin care as well.

That's pretty much my routine and I noticed the effects of wrinkles and other skin imperfections improved and I appeared and felt younger. So, give it a try!

The last thing I will mention before we go to the next chapter is to reiterate the importance of staying hydrated. I'm basically going to repeat what I mentioned in *Chapter 3* in case you missed it (in italics – so if you read *Chapter 3* you can skip this) ...

One other point. Since our bodies are made up of a lot of water, I recommend that you drink a lot of it. How much you ask? Most people would say 8 eight-ounce glasses a day (total of 8 x 8 = 64 ounces per day). I never liked that answer. I just can't believe the water need is the same for a 90-pound female gymnast as it is for a 250-pound male body builder. It obviously depends on your weight and activity level. As a rule of thumb, I like to take my weight and multiply by 2/3 to come up with the total ounces to drink per day. For me it would be 150 lbs. x 2/3 = 100 ounces a day. The average bottle of water has about 16 ounces in it so about six of those bottles a day would be right for me. I also will add an additional twelve ounces for every thirty minutes of working out on top of that. I learned these tidbits from the article that can be found here from Slender Kitchen: http://www.slenderkitchen.com/article/how-to-calculate-how-much-water-you-should-drink-a-day.

There are other sites on the Internet that will recommend anywhere from ½ ounce to 1 full ounce of water per day per body weight. I would experiment to see what works well for you. The 2/3 version works for me. I would start there and then modify for what works for you.

To make it easier, I have water bottles everywhere. One on a table next to my bed, one in my basement where I work out, one in my office next to my computer, one in both of my cars, one on the table in the family room where I watch television. That's seven bottles of water spread out around my house and cars! I also always use filtered water so I'm not getting all the impurities from tap water and filtered water just tastes better. I also carry around a large Hydro Flask (basically a big metal can) almost everywhere I go so I have no excuse to not get the water in.

Just be prepared to pee – I mean A LOT! And I know this may be gross but a good indicator to see if you are well enough hydrated is to look at your pee. If it's clear like water with a very slight yellow color you are doing well. If it's darker yellow, then drink some water and if it's brown stop everything and drink a lot of water! If it's completely clear (not likely) like water with absolutely no yellow hue you are probably overdoing the drinking a bit. A great chart can be found in this article from the Cleveland Clinic: https://health.clevelandclinic.org/2013/10/what-the-color-of-your-urine-says-about-you-infographic/.

So enough about reducing wrinkles and imperfections of the skin. Let's move on … time to get fit!

5 - Keeping fit and working out

Since I was a teenager, I always saw the importance to include aerobic and resistance training into my daily routine (this is especially important as you age so you don't lose muscle and gain excessive fat). After all, you want to be able to walk when you are in your golden years!

From my research, it seems that most of us should be getting in at least 30 to 60 minutes of exercise a day. Now you can join a gym, I'm not going to say no to that, and there are some great reasons to join a gym, but I went the route of utilizing the Internet to get in most of my workouts. The exception is running and only because running alone, or inside, is not fun for me. I like to make running social. More on running later. Back to resistance workouts.

There is a great site that offers you the ability to workout at home and get it done fast and efficiently. That being said, this works for me, but if you are the type that can't motivate yourself to push play on the exercise videos and do the workout, then a personal trainer or a good gym that provides that motivation may be what you need. After all, we are all different and there isn't one solution for everyone. The most important point is to make sure we are all getting the workouts in consistently and we are changing up the workouts to get the most out of them. Basically spending 30 minutes a day on the elliptical isn't the way to go.

I used to own a running store called *Fleet Feet*. It's a franchise and I owned the one in Gaithersburg, Maryland for thirteen years before I handed it off to some great new owners. You can find these stores nationwide at www.fleetfeet.com.

I was lucky. Through the store, I met many others who ran and that enabled me to run with a group of people or with my wife who also runs. This really helped motivate me for the runs. That was my major source of cardio since I really can't stand the treadmill and you will probably never see me on an elliptical. Unless it's on an Elliptigo®. Don't know what an Elliptigo® is? It's basically an elliptical that rides like a bike outside. You can see it here: https://www.elliptigo.com

It may be great to complete your cardio indoors but I love the outdoors and running with others. I also am not a fan of running alone so running with a group of positive minded individuals really helped me. It actually made running fun!

Fleet Feet stores nationwide as well as other running stores offer free fun runs and paid training programs for specific races or events. It's a fun way to stay healthy and meet new people and have a lot of fun. I definitely recommend finding a running store near you and give it a try. What do you have to lose? You may end up meeting life-long friends in the process and add a new dimension to your life!

This now brings us back to resistance training. There is a great source of workout videos on www.beachbody.com. There are many different types of workouts to choose from.   I personally enjoy weightlifting or some type of functional fitness.

I was first introduced to these videos from an instructor named Tony Horton (not in person but from the Internet). This dude can be extreme but what I really liked about his P90X series videos (and he has other less extreme routines as well) is that you can modify them so if you can't keep up with what his crazies are doing on your first day of playing the video then you can do a more moderate version. Then as you progress you can start to do the more extreme versions of the exercises. If you are already working out then you should be able to jump right in. So I am listing on the next page the videos I have completed since writing this book (all are on www.Beachbody.com):

Program	Instructor	Comments
P90X	Tony Horton	A great introduction to functional fitness and a way to get your butt kicked (but in a good way). Expect over an hour each workout. Workouts are about one hour.
P90X2	Tony Horton	Focused on strength and balancing – I couldn't do this one completely, I'm not coordinated enough.
P90X3	Tony Horton	Agility and strength – only 30 minute workouts.
P90	Tony Horton	A great workout for beginners – about 30 minutes per workout.
21 Day Fix	Autumn Calabrese	30 minute cardio and weightlifting workouts with nutrition guidelines.
Body Beast	Sagi Kalev	30 – 50 minute workouts with heavy weightlifting.
The Master's Hammer & Chisel	Autumn Calabrese & Sagi Kalev	Great workouts that focus on body sculpting (Chisel) and bodybuilding (Hammer).
Shift Shop	Chris Downing	About 40 minutes with cardio and resistance training.
Liift4	Joel Freeman	About 40 minutes of lifting, hiit (cardio) and core exercises.
Tony Horton's 10 Minute Workout	Tony Horton	A selection of workouts that work all the muscles. Each video lasts 10 minutes and you can do multiple workouts in a day.

These are some of the workouts that work for me. I mix them up so I'm not doing the same thing over and over again. I've also done other workouts but these are the ones that I either liked the best or that were more memorable. And when I say that, I have to admit that some of these workouts I didn't like so much when I was doing them (I would actually cuss at the trainer on the screen knowing full well they couldn't hear me) but was very glad I did the workouts. The results were great and that's what really matters.

I continue doing these workouts even today. By mixing up the workouts, I am getting the benefit of *muscle confusion*. Basically, the muscles don't become used to doing the same thing every day and not progressing. It's also more fun because I'm not doing the same thing day in and day out and growing tired of it. Because of this I am more likely to keep up with the workouts.

Hence why I make fun of the elliptical machine. Your body can't change if that's all you do but many people fall into that as their only workout.

Not a good idea!

As I mentioned previously, I also run about three miles, three to four times a week. I run at a pace that I can easily have a discussion with the person, or people, I'm running with. That way I know I'm not running too fast. This keeps me injury free and from completely loathing the workout. If that happens, then I either have to stop or I want to stop, and that's not a good thing.

I believe the combination of the aerobic (running) and the resistance training (the workouts mentioned above) do a great job in keeping me as fit as I can be without overdoing it. But just because these work for me they may not be the best for you.

Please look at the www.Beachbody.com workouts, local gyms, personal trainers, Cross-fit gyms, yoga studios, functional fitness gyms, running and walking groups, etc. in your own communities and find routines that work for you. Just keep in mind a balance of cardio and resistance training would be the way to go. And don't think you are too old to start. Check with your doctors and see if they have any concerns, but most doctors I've dealt with believe their patients should work out more than they do. In general we live a very sedimentary life-style and that is not good in the long run. That's why you see sixty-year olds barely able to walk and, in contrast, people in their 90's actually running marathons (yes all 26.2 miles)!

Another point I'd like to bring up. I hear this many, many times (especially from women) but don't worry about getting *too big*. I hate to burst your bubble but it's not going to happen. It will take a lot more then what I'm showing you in this book to be a professional body builder so don't think you will get huge doing these routines.

I'm going to pick on women here for a moment (sorry about that) but a lot of women are afraid to lift weights because they believe they will become too muscular and look like a man. Don't worry, you won't. I must warn you, however, if you perform these workouts you probably will get into the best physical shape in your life and look like a genuine hottie!

The other thing I get in everyday (or at least five to seven times a week) is a quick ten to twenty minute yoga workout. This is probably one of the most important activities I do for my health and keeping as young as possible.

I started the practice of yoga out of fear. I was first introduced to it from Tony Horton on his P90x routine. So, what was I afraid of? From owning the running store, I would see all types of customers. Some appeared much older than their age and I remember seeing individuals as young as 50 years old barely able to walk. They were stiff, and some walked bent over with a cane almost having to look at the floor. They couldn't stand up straight!

I was terrified of becoming like that as I aged. I was never that flexible my whole life, but I felt myself becoming even stiffer as I aged. I could barely touch my shins in a forward fold. I knew I had to do something to change this.

So, I checked out yoga routines (the routines in the P90x series are hard to do but can be modified). I will list some other, more beginner options, below, but I want to point out that I can now touch the floor in a forward fold and some of the other poses: upward dog (or full cobra), downward dog, cat/cow, mountain, plank, child's, twists: all have helped me tremendously in my flexibility and just the way I walk. I actually look taller now than I did years ago because my posture is so much better. I highly recommend everyone do yoga at least 4 times a week.

Some routines other than those related to the P90X series that I've found on youtube are here:

Yoga   by   Candice
(https://www.youtube.com/user/YOGABYCANDACE)

   – 20   min   yoga   flow   for   beginners   at
https://www.youtube.com/watch?v=BdTzZuwGEOw

Yoga by Candice (https://www.youtube.com/user/YOGABYCANDACE)

– *20 minute total body beginner flow* at https://www.youtube.com/watch?v=h0Qeu8KX1BE&t=243s

Boho Beautiful (https://www.youtube.com/channel/UCWN2FPlvg9r-LnUyepH9IaQ)

– *Easy Yoga for Beginners ❤Full Body Gentle Flow* at https://www.youtube.com/watch?v=3_Q-yYfjeBM

Yoga with Adriene (https://www.youtube.com/channel/UCFKE7WVJfvaHW5q283SxchA)

– *Yoga For Complete Beginners – 20 Minute Home Yoga Workout!* at: https://www.youtube.com/watch?v=v7AYKMP6rOE.

SaraBethYoga (https://www.youtube.com/channel/UC-0CzRZeML8zw4pFTVDq65Q)

– *20 Minute Yoga for Complete Beginners | Easy Stretching* at https://www.youtube.com/watch?v=_2PB4J5h7bI

SaraBethYoga (https://www.youtube.com/channel/UC-0CzRZeML8zw4pFTVDq65Q)

- *10 minute Morning Yoga for Beginners* at https://www.youtube.com/watch?v=VaoV1PrYft4

SaraBethYoga (https://www.youtube.com/channel/UC-0CzRZeML8zw4pFTVDq65Q)

– 10 Minute Simple Yoga Flow | SarahBethYoga at https://www.youtube.com/watch?v=t3joHNOOyYY

SaraBethYoga (https://www.youtube.com/channel/UC-0CzRZeML8zw4pFTVDq65Q)

– 10 minute Simple Slow Stretch Yoga (all levels!) | Yoga for Beginners at https://www.youtube.com/watch?v=_0xZ3iOswYM

TOGATX (https://www.youtube.com/channel/UCAwPqAM_ONIyl1EHU5hDe4Q)

– Morning Yoga - 10 Minute Stretch & Strengthen Sequence at https://www.youtube.com/watch?v=2c_oijA34Z8.

These are some of the videos I like the best when looking on www.youtube.com. I'm sure there are many more that I didn't list – there are many out there and all for free!

As I mentioned above I also do the yoga routines from P90X, P90X2 & P90X3 and other yoga routines on www.beachbody.com but the yoga routines on www.beachbody.com are between thirty minutes to an hour so they are a bit longer than the www.youtube.com videos I mentioned above.

If you are interested, try these out and then check out others. If you are new to yoga, I would recommend starting with a 10 minute beginner routine, do that for a week or so, and then move up from there. Have fun with it.

There are some really great instructors on the Internet that have some great content. Once again, to do yoga from watching a video you have to have the discipline to turn on your computer and do the routines.

69

If you have a hard time doing that then I would suggest finding a yoga instructor and class in your local area that can provide you the motivation and also be there to correct your moves and postures to make sure you are doing the yoga moves right. Just like the running groups, finding a local class will also open the doors to meet other individuals that share your goal of living a more positive, productive and happier life. Who knows, you might meet your best friend there!

Just please give yoga a try, you won't regret it. It may be a little painful during the practice but it is so refreshing afterwards and you will feel great walking around with fantastic posture that will keep you young as you age.

One other note before we leave this chapter. I'm going to stress not to overdue these workouts. Don't think you should increase the weight every day or feel that you have to up the miles or speed during your runs every day. That's a great way to get hurt or burned out to the point you stop working out altogether. Have fun with the workouts and always feel you can do a little more after the workout.

A lot of trainers will disagree with me on this and want you to be totally spent after the workout but I want you to keep it going for the rest of your life and not quit. Just remember why you started working out in the first place. If your goal is to stay young and healthy then have fun with it and don't push so hard that you quit in the long-term. It should be a lifestyle – your journey for a healthier, happier more youthful life. If your goal is to win a body building contest or win the Boston Marathon then by all means listen to your coach. But most of us are not training for a professional team or the Olympics so be reasonable in your workouts. It's not about getting hurt or burned out. It's about a healthy lifestyle that you can live with forever.

Most personal trainers would prefer you to lower the weight and use great form than to use bad form and use too much weight. One way will deliver great results and the other a trip to the doctor's office.

Also, please don't stress over the workouts and have fun with them. Do the best you can and modify if you have to. Don't feel if you miss a workout it's the end of the world. It's okay. Life gets in the way at times and this is nothing to get stressed about. Just do your best. As I mentioned before, my goal is to workout with resistance training four to five times a week and run three to four times a week. Yoga every day. If I shoot for that then I usually will get 80% to 100% done. What would I accomplish if I didn't have this goal? Probably not as much as I do get done.

Also, concentrate on what you do and not what you don't do. You will feel better if you do. Instead of saying: *Man, I had an okay week but I missed my Thursday run*, say: *I killed it this week! Hit the weights four days and ran two! Also did four yoga sessions. I ROCKED IT! I am proud of myself.*

I mean, which one of these would you prefer to tell yourself?

So, I encourage you to make working out a priority, do your best during the workouts, set your goals realistically high and honestly do your best to hit those goals. But don't beat yourself up if you fall a little short. As long as you really do try your best you can't feel bad.

I know I'm going to beat this point into the ground but be sure to pick routines that you honestly feel you can do your whole life. Looking and feeling years younger is a journey to the *Fountain of Youth* that you should continue until the day you die. Your quality of life will be greatly improved if you do!

And you will be richer than Ponce de Leon, or any other treasure hunter, if you accomplish these workouts because you will have the greatest gift of all. The gift of great health!

Chapter 6 - What you put in your stomach really does matter

I'm going to get this out right now. Initially you probably won't like me. But when you follow my suggestions and look and feel years younger you will then show me the love.

But before we get to the bad news, I want to let you know my philosophy on diets and why I think most people fail on them. First of all, you have to stop thinking about diets as what you *can't* eat or limiting what you eat. This only leads the mind to feel it's depriving the body. You have to think more about what *SHOULD* I be eating. Remember, the physical reason why we eat is to get the right balance of nutrients to keep the body and mind healthy. Starving yourself is not the answer.

Somewhere we really messed up the reason why we need to eat with the introduction of fast food, preservatives, artificial flavors, processed sugar, flour etc. What were we thinking? Do we really think a frosted pop-tart in the toaster oven is a good way for our kids to start the day? I've seen adults at work bringing their breakfast in with them. A box of donuts and a mega-sized cola with all the added caffeine and processed sugar. Why do we reward our children with candy, cakes and fast food? Instilling life-long desires for something they shouldn't be eating in the first place. That's why we crave this junk, it's been implanted in us since childhood.

Does this even make sense? Why would we do that to ourselves? No wonder those diagnosed with diabetes and obesity is at epic levels and still rising. That's why most Americans and Europeans are classified as obese. The body was never meant to take in that much sugar and processed garbage.

Did you know that according to the United States Department of Agriculture (USDA) that the average American consumes 150 to 170 pounds of sugar per year? That's just an average so some individuals consume a whopping 300 or more pounds of sugar per year. To put this in perspective, in the early 1800's that average was 4 to 6 pounds a year. So, on average we are consuming about 30 times more sugar now then we were just a couple of centuries ago! A great article on this can be found here in this Bamboocore Fitness article: *Not So Sweet – The Average American Consumes 150-170 Pounds Of Sugar Each Year* at: https://bamboocorefitness.com/not-so-sweet-the-average-american-consumes-150-170-pounds-of-sugar-each-year/. This surprises me because shouldn't we be learning more about nutrition and health and getting better instead of going backwards? What's that all about?

Somehow, we have allowed big business to convince us that their unhealthy products are actually good for us. An example are fruit rolls. Somehow these treats are pushed off as a healthy alternative to candy. Have you actually read the label on fruit rolls? Not exactly a health food after all.

In this Wikipedia content: *Fruit Roll-Ups* (https://en.wikipedia.org/wiki/Fruit_Roll-Ups) it states that the main ingredient in fruit roll-ups is sugar. In fact, five different types of sugar: sugar from pear juice concentrate, corn syrup, dried corn syrup, sugar, and dextrose. They also contain small amounts of partially hydrogenated cottonseed oil, citric acid, sodium citrate, acetylated monoglycerides, fruit pectin, malic acid, ascorbic acid, natural flavors, and artificial colors.

Is this really healthier than candy?

We need to expose this whole idea of what is considered healthy and what is not if we truly want to look and feel years younger and just live happier, healthier lives.

So, the bad news (although I really think its good news): If you want to live a healthy, happier life, you need to take all processed foods out of your diet. Period! This means no sodas, chips, bags of cookies, fruit rolls, crackers, pretzels, fast food, etc. Look for wholesome organic foods and shop smarter. You will be happy with the result!

A lot of people tell me they can't help themselves from snacking on these products. It's right in front of them and they just eat it. Here is a suggestion: don't buy this crap! Eating healthy always starts at the grocery store.

Here's a great tip. Don't go to the grocery store when you are hungry – not a good idea. If you do go to the grocery store hungry, you probably will purchase junk you just don't need. Remember, if the bag of cookies or candy is not in your house, you can't reach for it because it's not there.

I've also heard time and time again from individuals that they purchase the cookies, candy and chips for their kids, then see the treats in the pantry and can't help themselves and nibble on one.

Or two, or three ...

I have an answer for you. Do yourself and your child a favor and don't buy the crap. Replace them with healthy organic snacks. They do exist. Visit the organic section of your grocery store, stay away from sugar, gluten and dairy and pick out some healthier treats.

As an example, you can replace a bag of Cheetos® cheese flavored chemistry lab experiment with an organic *Please Peas*™ and be much better off. What are *Please Peas*™ you ask? They look like green Cheetos®, taste great (at least I think so) and are much better for you. The great thing is that they are made out of organic peas and not toxic orange waste. Here is a www.youtube.com review of it by Gluten Free Discoveries (https://www.youtube.com/channel/UCWL2tmKP8hCgZZvO5faN9Rw) at *Peeled Snacks Peas Please Taste Test & Review! | Gluten Free Discoveries* (https://www.youtube.com/watch?v=dYOOhetoRSc).

Better yet, grab a carrot or a banana or some type of raw whole food. Your body will be glad you did.

I also want to say that you can reward yourself with dessert or another favorite dish if you want. I would suggest making that organic as well and stay away from dairy & gluten products as much as you can, but it's okay to indulge a little and have that organic gluten-free chocolate chip cookie after dinner. Just not a whole bag of them! And I also want to say that it's okay to cheat once in a while. If I've been good all week, I feel it's okay to go out to dinner on the weekend. I still make better choices, but I allow myself to cheat occasionally. We are human after all!

Getting back to my journey to the *Fountain of Youth* and my ride through the Internet to look and feel years younger, there are a few websites that can help. I'll get to those in a minute. Unfortunately, what I found about *diet*, and diets in general, is that there are several different points of view on the subject. Vegan, vegetarian, pescatarian, paleo, gluten-free, dairy free, keto, intermittent fasting, eating every 2 ½ hours, etc.

The options are infinite and it can make your head spin just trying to figure it all out. On top of that not all philosophies of diet work for everyone. Some of us have food allergies or can handle certain foods better than others. It can be quite overwhelming!

What I find works for me and what I endorse is a diet of organic foods, no preservatives, high in protein, good carbs (but stay away from gluten and sugar) lots of vegetables, some fruits, not much dairy. A good article on the subject can be found in this Muscle and Fitness (https://www.muscleandfitness.com) website and helps with good meal ideas: *The Beginner Bodybuilder's 4-Week Meal Plan* at http://www.muscleandfitness.com/nutrition/meal-plans/beginner-bodybuilder-s-4-week-meal-plan.

If you continue through the article it also has suggestions for meals here: *The Beginner Bodybuilder's 4-Week Meal Plan* at http://www.muscleandfitness.com/nutrition/meal-plans/beginner-bodybuilder-s-4-week-meal-plan?page=2.

One note I would make. They suggest more dairy then I would recommend. I also typically substitute almond milk for regular milk. If I do consume dairy products I tend to have either plain organic Greek yogurt or kefir. I'll add organic raw honey to it to make it taste like a treat! But this is a personal decision so if you like milk and you don't suffer any side effects then go for it.

I also prefer eating many small meals a day versus just three large ones, but that's just me. This way I can get more great nutrients in and keep my body fueled all day long. It also curbs my desire to snack on junk food. If I get in all my nutrient dense meals I really don't want to eat anything else.

I typically eat every 2 ½ to 3 hours. This way my body has constant nourishment and I can get into fat burn mode. The trick is to keep it there so if you go this route, just like everything else, consistency is the key.

There is a small article on what Tony Horton (P90X series extreme workout creator – www.tonyhortonlife.com) eats in a day right here: *This is the carefully planned diet of celebrity trainer Tony Horton* by Matt Johnston: http://www.businessinsider.com/tony-hortons-diet-and-nutrition-2015-5. Doesn't sound that bad, right? And he doesn't mention it, but knowing Tony Horton, I believe it's either all or mostly organic.

Another good article on healthy eating can be found here: *Eat to Feel Young:*   http://www.tonyhortonlife.com/post/2016/3/17/eat-to. Again, lean protein is important. Vegetables and fruits should be eaten daily. Stay away from processed foods and eat real food. Look at the ingredients of some of the products you find in the supermarket. Stay away from those that have ingredients you can't pronounce or have no idea what it is.

I would also try to take out as much gluten from your diet as you can. Gluten products such as wheat (bread, crackers, white flour and pasta) can cause inflammation and are hard to digest. A great list of foods to avoid and foods to eat can be found in this great Healthline (www.healthline.com) article I found during my journey: *Gluten Intolerance Food List: What to Avoid and What to Eat:* http://www.healthline.com/health/allergies/gluten-food-list#overview1. A lot of these foods are processed and don't give you the nutrients you need but just fill you up with empty carbs that will eventually be stored as fat. These products can also cause inflammation in the body and cause all sorts of issues you just don't want or need.

Another article I'll mention is from Dr. Oz (yes the guy with the television show): *JJ Smiths 10-Day Tummy Detox Plan to eliminate constipation & bloating and improve gut & digestive health:* http://s.doctoroz.com/Tummy-Detox-One-Sheet-v3.jpg. This is meant for detoxing the stomach but not only helps to flatten out the tummy (who doesn't want that) but also is just a great guide on how to shop and eat a lot healthier.

This brings me to another point. Try to find time to cook. What's great about cooking your own meals is that you control what goes into them. If you pick out (remember all organic) skinless chicken breast (if not organic then at least grass-fed, free range, hormone free) put some good organic spices on it, cook up an organic sweet potato (with some cinnamon) and add an organic salad with spinach, kale, cherry tomatoes, cucumber, red pepper, carrots, celery, mushrooms and onions, then you have a very healthy meal with lean protein, good carbs, low fat, filled with vitamins, without preservatives, artificial colors or artificial dyes and your body, hair, face, skin and mind will thank you.

You can always switch out the chicken protein with fish, lean beef, turkey or your favorite vegetarian or vegan protein. You can also switch out the starch, so instead of a sweet potato you can have brown rice or quinoa. You can switch the salad for mixed vegetables, broccoli, or asparagus. This way you can have a lot of different meals with the same idea in mind: a lean protein, a good gluten free carb and a vegetable.

Another great www.youtube.com video channel I came across in my journey to the *Fountain of Youth* is from Dr. Mona Vand, a pharmacist. Her Youtube channel can be found here: https://www.youtube.com/channel/UC0GkEyks1Nnzhsi9bCZTIjA. She has some great videos on eating healthy, especially if you want to go the vegan route like she does. She not only discusses good food choices but the best time to eat them. So as you become more sophisticated in what you eat you can work out when you eat these products. I tend not to mix too many carbs and proteins anymore (unless I'm in my bulk phase –

more on that later) to aid in digestion and I try to eat my fruit in the morning, then progress to heavier meals as the day goes on. I know this is different than a lot of opinions out there, but I think she has something here.

A great video on food combinations by Dr. Mona Vand is here: *Food Combining Basics (2017) | Dr Mona Vand:* https://www.youtube.com/watch?v=nmu6hJJdSe4 (part one) and: *Food Combining Basics Part 2 (2018) | Dr Mona Vand:* https://www.youtube.com/watch?v=WRnG9Ay3ywQ. She also has other helpful videos on heathy snacks, what she eats for breakfast, lunch & dinner, face massage and masks and other helpful healthy tips.

Another tip -- drink a lot of water during the day but not with your meals. Several sites have stated that you need your stomach acids at their best when digesting food so 20 minutes before, during and about 20 minutes after a meal, try not to drink too much water. Water will dilute the stomach acids and they won't be as effective in breaking down the food. If you don't digest food well then you don't get the full benefit of nutrient absorption and the food starts to decompose in your intestines and causes gas and bloating.

Make sure to chew your food well before swallowing. The more you chew your food the easier it will be digested, and nutrients absorbed by the body.

During the rest of the day drink up that water!

Because water is probably the most important single part of health, I mention it a few times in this book. So if you read some of the other chapters I'm going to warn you now that the next several paragraphs will be a repeat of what I stated earlier. I have the section in italics in case you already read this and want to skip it.

Here goes …

One other point. Since our bodies are made up of a lot of water, I recommend that you drink a lot of water. How much you ask? Most people would say 8 eight-ounce glasses a day (total of 8 x 8 = 64 ounces per day).

I never liked that answer.

I just can't believe the water need is the same for a 90-pound female gymnast as it is for a 250-pound male body builder. It obviously depends on your weight and activity level. As a rule of thumb, I like to take my weight and multiply by 2/3 to come up with the total ounces to drink per day. For me it would be 150 lbs. x 2/3 = 100 ounces a day. The average bottle of water has about sixteen ounces in it so a little more than six of those bottles a day would be right for me. I also will add an additional twelve ounces for every thirty minutes of working out on top of that. I learned these tidbits from the article that can be found here from Slender Kitchen: How to Calculate How Much Water You Should Drink A Day, by Kristen Mccaffrey at: http://www.slenderkitchen.com/article/how-to-calculate-how-much-water-you-should-drink-a-day.

There are other sites on the Internet that will recommend anywhere from ½ ounce to 1 full ounce of water per day per body weight.

I would experiment to see what works well for you. The 2/3 version works for me. I would start there and then modify for what works for you.

To make it easier, I have water bottles everywhere. One on a table next to my bed, one in my basement where I work out, one in my office next to my computer, one in both of my cars, one on the table in the family room where I watch television. That's seven bottles of water spread out around my house and cars! I also always use filtered water so I'm not getting all the impurities from tap water and filtered water just tastes better. I also carry around a large Hydro Flask® (basically a big metal can) almost everywhere I go so I have no excuse to get the water in. The other seven bottles are actually just for back up in case I don't have my Hydro Flask® with me.

Just be prepared to pee – I mean A LOT! And I know this may be gross but a good indicator to see if you are well enough hydrated is to inspect your pee. If it's clear like water with a very slight yellow hue you are doing great. If it's darker yellow, then drink some water and if it's brown stop everything and drink a lot of water! If it's completely clear (not likely) like water with absolutely no yellow hue you are probably overdoing the drinking a bit. A great chart can be found in this article from the Cleveland Clinic: What The Color of Your Urine Says About You: Color, density, and smell can reveal health problems at: https://health.clevelandclinic.org/2013/10/what-the-color-of-your-urine-says-about-you-infographic/.

I also have a glass or two of red wine (at dinner or socially) about once a week. You don't have to do this but I like it and you must live a little. Again, we are human, after all, and not machines. I used to have a glass or two every night but that was too much alcohol and sugar consumption for me. So now I limit the alcohol to one to two glasses per week (sometimes less). I probably would be better off not having any alcohol at all but I am only human! Everyone has to make their own decision whether to include alcohol in their diets but I would recommend limiting it to a couple of drinks a week. Alcohol is very dehydrating and has a lot of sugar in it, so eliminate or limit your intake.

A basic day of my diet would include the following:

Morning:

- Small amount of warm water with powdered collagen (1 & 3) supplement, juice from a lemon, tablespoon of organic apple cider vinegar.
- Vitamins (all natural): multi-vitamin, D3, C (with rose hips), tart cherry & E (so five separate pills).
- Tablespoon each (all organic) of fish oil & olive oil.
- Smoothie to include (all organic) coconut water, spinach, kale, blueberries, raspberries, blackberries, strawberries, golden berries, turmeric (fresh not powder), ginger (fresh not powder), walnuts, almonds, multi-nut spread, ½ scoop of Shakeology®, scoop of whey unsweetened protein powder & lemon juice from ½ lemon.
- Organic oatmeal with either organic peanut butter or organic multi-nut butter.

- Organic Matcha green tea with organic raw honey, organic and unrefined coconut oil & organic cinnamon.
- About once a week I'll replace the smoothie and oatmeal with eggs. Five to six eggs if I'm in my bulking phase and two to three in my cutting phase (more on bulking and cutting phase at the end of the chapter). I'll also add a piece of Ezekiel Bread.

After Workout:

- Smoothie to include, yes I know this is crazy so you don't have to go overboard like this: (once again all of this is organic): almond milk, spinach, kale, carrots, celery, cucumber, onion, red peppers, cherry tomatoes, mushrooms, sweet potatoes (raw), avocado, turmeric (fresh not powder), ginger (fresh not powder), multi-nut butter, scoop of Shakeology®, scoop of unsweetened whey protein powder. Typically I will make three of these at a time in the blender and have them for three days. So I triple the amounts for the Shakeology® and unsweetened whey protein powder.

Afternoon Snack:

- Some sort of organic & gluten-free protein bar. I like the gomacro® protein replenishment bars (https://www.gomacro.com) the best (either with peanut butter or cashew butter) but if you are going to do this you need to find one you like. There are so many options of protein bars that it will literally make your head spin.

Lunch:

- Organic turkey slices with Ezekiel bread or
- Organic sardines or eggs
- Sometimes an organic salad

Before Dinner Snack:

- Handful of organic walnuts and almonds

Dinner:

- Lean organic chicken, beef or turkey.
- Organic sweet potato, quinoa with vegetables or rice with vegetables.
- Organic salad with spinach, kale, carrots, celery, cucumber, onion, red peppers, tomatoes, mushrooms.

Dessert:

- Organic 85% dark chocolate – 1 or 2 squares or a few dark chocolate covered almonds.

After Dinner Snack:

- Beef, Turkey & Chicken bone broth.
- Some sort of organic & gluten-free protein bar.

Right Before Bed:

- Some type of organic, vegan protein shake. I like the Orgain Organic Nutrition™ Vegan All-in-One Protein Shake (https://www.orgain.com/protein/nutrition-shakes/vegetarian-protein-shakes.html#851770003216).

Now this is a lot of food but I am trying to build muscle and gain weight (the right kind) so if that is not your goal you may want to change this up a bit. The good thing about eating this much, and all through the day, is that you are filling up with organic nutrient-dense foods that your body needs and keeps you full so you don't crave bad food. You just aren't hungry enough to eat the junk. But I guarantee that if you work out, get your sleep, and eat this way, you will lose fat and gain muscle. Isn't that the goal?

Now when I'm in crazy bulk phase (not often) I will also add three tablespoons of olive oil (in a shot glass) three times a day. Olive oil has 120 calories per tablespoon so that gives me an additional whopping 3 x 3 x 120 = 1,080 calories of a healthy fat every day! That will help pack on the quality muscle pounds! But I only do this for a short period (one or two weeks at most) because it is a bit hard on the body and even though it's a healthy fat, it is a fat and I wouldn't recommend this for everyone.

So I would like to take a little time to discuss the bulking and cutting phase of building a strong, sexy body. If you talk to a bodybuilder (male or female) they will probably tell you that it's very hard to put on muscle at the same time you are reducing fat. So what is the answer? A two phased cycle. So the first phase is bulk. This will help you gain big muscle while adding minimal dreaded fat but not nearly the amount of fat you would gain if you ate poorly. You do this for a few months until you are actually over the weight you want to end at. Then you cut the fat, carbs and total calories in your diet to reduce the fat.

This is the technique that many actors and actresses have used to get to their desired result. An example is what Chris Hemsworth does to get ready for a Thor movie. Other actors who have done this are: Mark Wahlberg (Pain & Gain), Chris Pratt (Guardians of the Galaxy), Chris Evans (Captain America), Hugh Jackman (Wolverine), Gal Gadot (Wonder Woman) & many others.

So, when implementing the bulk & cut phase diet with your resistance and cardio training, you need to have patience (just like everything else) to get to your desired build. There is a great video on regarding this from Celebrity Workout Routines (https://www.youtube.com/channel/UCUkV_XZUxiPyBrnP5Qme59A) called: *Mark   Wahlberg   Diet   Plan*   at: https://www.youtube.com/watch?v=XgNSky8TaEw.

From this video you can see the layout of the bulking/cutting phase. The actors mentioned above, as well as many others, all follow this same basic principle when getting their bodies in the best shape of their lives.

You can also see from the video that in the bulking phase you have to eat healthy foods, not junk. Otherwise you won't be fueling your muscles and you will only be putting on a lot of fat. Remember that, even though you are in bulk phase, you want to maximize muscle gain and minimize fat gain.

Another great video to watch so you can hear how this all works from the actors themselves can be found on this www.youtube.com video   from   fellow   youtuber   Radoslav   Detchev (https://www.youtube.com/channel/UCPKxSx5Zp0Lxv4CLP0t2GqA) called *Actors   Give   Advice   on   Diet   &   Exercise*   at: https://www.youtube.com/watch?v=rF3ixuORPaw&t=252s. Take a look. It's not only informational but quite interesting to hear the diet and workout plans these actors had to go through to look the part. After all, they are all human also and they aren't just blessed with being in great shape. They all had to work very hard to get there. It's not easy looking like a superhero. It takes patience, time and work. Sound familiar?

To simplify the equation of weight gain and weight loss, it really comes down to this. Calories consumed versus calories burned. So if you want to gain weight, you need to consume more calories than you burn. If you want to lose weight, you need to consume fewer calories than you burn. So how can you tell? You can either pick a diet and an exercise routine and watch what happens or you can be more scientific about it.

An example, let's say you want to lose weight. You go on a specific diet and workout program and in a week see if you lost weight. If you didn't, or worse you gained, then you need to reduce how many calories you take in. Adjust your diet for the next week and see what happens. Just make sure you are counting all your calories. Yes that cracker you snuck in right before bed when no one was looking counts!

A more scientific way to work this is to actually count all your calories. Look at the labels and write down what you eat or get an app on your phone (there are many out here). Get a fitness tracker and wear it all the time. It will estimate calories burned. If the calories you count up are more than what your fitness tracker says you are burning then you will gain weight. If the calories you count up are less than what your fitness tracker says you are burning then you will lose weight. Simple as that.

Google fitness trackers and calories counters and you will see there are many devices and apps available to accomplish this task. So many and so different I'm going to leave that as a homework project for you if you want to go that route.

I want to end, so this will be the real last note, with this advice: do not to beat yourself up if you slip occasionally. I mean if you go over to someone's house you should eat what they serve you! Right? Otherwise you won't get invited over anymore. Just make sure when you are over there to make the best choices available to you. Don't eat the bread, stick with the lean protein, and eat just a few carbs. You don't have to let someone else dictate your total health choices, but there are ways to satisfy them without destroying your diet.

Or if you go out on your birthday to that fancy restaurant – eat up! I know I do. Just make a real honest effort to follow these diet guidelines and if you achieve 80% - 90% of the plan then you are much, much better than the average person and you, and everyone else, will notice that difference as well!

Now with this said, if you are working with a health coach or a doctor on your diet, please listen to them before listening to me. Don't sabotage your hard work based on what I'm saying above. I don't want your coaches or doctors coming after me! So listen to them first.

Now on to a healthy, happy mind …

Chapter 7 - The body cannot live without the mind

The body cannot live without the mind. I heard that first (or something like it) from a movie called *The Matrix.* I have to say that was a strange but brilliant movie. But the quote is very true. In order to look and feel years younger I knew I needed to make my mind right. This is no easy task. The problem is, most of us don't have our mind right.

There are a few ways I found that helped me achieve a healthy mind and hopefully they will help you as well. One, I am the kind of person that has to have goals and I actually have to believe I can achieve the goals I set for myself. Basically, I would never grow my hair back, reduce wrinkles, and get into great shape and look and feel years younger unless I believed that I could.

Period!

So, if you aren't going to believe that you can achieve these amazing results and that this book is full of crap, then you might as well give up now. Because, as I mentioned before, to grow your hair, reduce your wrinkles and get into the best shape of your life is going to take work, time and patience. You will not notice results immediately nor will you notice changes every day, so, if you don't believe that you will change in the long-term, then you will most likely give up and not accomplish your goal to look and feel years younger. Believe in the process and in yourself and you will get there. It's just a matter of time. And if you take the amount of time compared to how long you lived, it's not that long.

So how do we believe in our goals? I actually pray for them daily. Now you may or may not believe in a higher being, which is up to you obviously, but if you want to achieve something you don't have yet, you need to convince yourself every day that you can achieve your goals. Whether it be that dream job, the returned affection of your crush, learning a new language, getting that degree, building muscle, losing weight, writing that next great novel, winning that race, reducing wrinkles, or just taking years off your looks and living a healthier, happier life!

I remember reading a book about *The Beatles* several years ago. From the book I learned that before *The Beatles* were famous, their leader, John Lennon, would ask the other members of the Fab 4 a couple of questions which he expected the same response. He would ask: *"Where are we going?"* The other members of *The Beatles* would shout: *"To the top!"* John would then shout: *"What top?"* and *The Beatles* would scream: *"To the very top!"*

The point is they believed from the very beginning that they would be the most famous rock group in history. They believed in themselves when they were a little-known English band playing in small venues in Germany and Liverpool. Barely anyone in the world knew who they were but that didn't matter to them. Even at that point they knew where they were heading. And I believe I can say with ease that *The Beatles* became the most famous and successful rock group of all time! In other words they went *to the very top!*

So, the number one rule is to honestly believe you will accomplish your goals and you will. Don't believe in them and the opposite will hold true.

A great book to read is: *The Secret* by Rhonda Byrne. You can get an idea what the book is about from here: http://www.thesecret.tv/. You can either believe that the universe is in place for us and we can use it to get what we desire for our life or you can choose not to believe. That's up to you. What I think, is if you follow the principles in the book, you will dream what you want, and you will achieve it because the more you believe in reaching your dreams, the more you will work towards those dreams. I probably sound like a nut but it does work. Don't believe me, give it a try!

Remember Martin Luther King Junior's famous speech: *"I have a dream …"* Every great leader, every highly successful person, has a dream first before achieving their goals. They will actually picture themselves achieving that goal every day. That's what keeps them focused. In order to obtain your goals, whatever they are, you will need to do the same.

What else can I tell you to help you get your mind right? I guess I'll just get to it. You must be positive. There I've said it. Just give it a try. You must work at this, but you need to take out all the negativity and hate in your life. As hard and painful as it may be you need to forgive everyone who has crossed you. That doesn't mean you have to hang out with them, but you must be bigger than them and take the high road. Don't wish then ill-will. That will only come back to haunt you. Forgive them and then don't cross paths with them if future meetings will bring up the same negativity and hate. Just know that some people are incompatible and that's okay. Just move on to bigger and better things. You deserve the best that life has to offer, right? Why complicate it any more than it has to be. As painful as it may be in the beginning, just remove yourself from negative people.

To have this positive mindset is easier said than done but you need to strive to do it. A great video on this is from Olgatoja (yes, the young lady with the facial massage exercises has a great video at this website): *Crystal Clear & Glowing Skin Tips (IT'S NOT WHAT YOU THINK) | PART 2:* https://www.youtube.com/watch?v=r0FtDQw5ADs (don't let the title fool you).

Now just to let you know this is harder than it seems. At least for me. I have to admit I struggle at this, but I do my best to conquer my anger at others and to learn to love everyone in the world. After all they are just people like you and me. Again, that doesn't mean I have to spend time with them (and it probably is better not to if they bring out negativity in your life) but it does mean not to dwell on what you don't like about them and just get past anything that will bring on negative thoughts. Frankly, you just don't need to pollute your mind with this non-productive crud that will just bring you down and crush your goals. Better to eliminate those from your life that are negative towards you and fill in with those that will support you and bring joy to your life.

Another thing I'll mention in this chapter is to allow yourself to be spiritual. This means different things to different people. I was raised Christian and I do pray to God every day. Basically to thank God for the great gift of a blessed life. This doesn't mean you must or have to have the same god. My wife is Jewish and I respect her religion and she respects mine. You need to choose what works for you. Maybe it's Buddha, Ganesh, Jesus or the God of Abraham or just a belief in self-awareness and the power of the positive mind or the power of the universe, but I do believe if you have a spiritual side to your life it helps you stay relaxed, joyful and young.

As I mentioned earlier in this book, I practice yoga almost every day. Yoga is a spiritual practice that has great physical benefits. In my case I do it to stay flexible, improve posture and calm myself down.

At the end of the yoga session it's customary for the trainer to say *Namaste*. The word is Hindu influenced and I've heard a few different literal translations but basically it means: *The light in me sees and respects the light in you.* In other words, we can be different, have different beliefs, but we are still all human and should respect and treat each other with respect.

If only everyone in the world felt this way. It would be a much better world where we are all truly created equal. But enough preaching (sorry about that)!

This brings me to meditation. You may think its way out there but I do believe it helps in relaxing the mind and the body. And in a good way.

A great site to learn the basics of meditation can be found here *How to Meditate* at: http://how-to-meditate.org/. You can also just perform an Internet search on meditation and you will find a wealth of information on the subject.

My biggest point here is that practicing meditation can help you relax and more importantly help you become more positive and, therefore, help you achieve your goals. It's a great way to erase the negativity in your life and see the best in everything. Not a bad thing! And you don't have to sit on top of a mountain, barefoot in a robe with the monks, and do it for days on end. You can actually practice meditation for five to ten minutes at a time in the comfort of your own home. That's what I do. Any more than that and my mind starts to wander. With practice you can increase the time.

I personally like the breathing or the mantra versions of meditation. During this time, you are concentrating on your breathing or you are concentrating on a single word (a mantra). This mantra should have no meaning to you. Like let's take a word like: *ing*. It doesn't mean anything. Just close your eyes, concentrate on your breathing then think the word *ing* or whatever mantra you chose, over and over again. A popular mantra is *om* – pronounced: a-u-m. Om is said to be the first sound heard at the creation of the universe.

While doing this you should start to relax. Your mind will probably start to stray away, but try your best to get back to your word. It takes practice and patience to do this. I still have a hard time with it. I chock that up to my ADD (or do I have ADHD)? I can't remember but I probably have one of those because my mind wanders everywhere!

Just like everything else, you will get better at meditation over time if you practice it nearly every day. Don't worry if it's hard at first. It's hard for everyone at first. That meeting or project you have coming up or that math test on Friday will always start to come into play. So, if you start to drift, pull it back. But please don't get frustrated or beat yourself up over this. The whole point is to relax your mind, not bring you more anguish. You probably have enough of that as it is. I know I do.

You will find if you can eliminate stress in your life, eliminate the negativity, increase the positivity, learn to love others and yourself, set your mind at peace, then your body will react to it. You will be a better person and you will physically look and feel better as well.

One other observation I've had in seeing how people age differently is that those who age slower tend to have more fun in their life. They learn to play and not just work all the time. They smile more, tend to be more friendly and accepting of others, and just all around more likeable. It's easy to get caught up in a cycle of waking up, going to work, driving home, blowing the horn and cursing at the dude who cut you off on the highway, taking care of the kids, eating dinner, and then going to bed. Only to do the same thing the next day. Not much of a life. Why live like that?

Remember to let yourself play a little each day and try to get out and do fun things, like you did when you were a child. Do this more often and you will find yourself becoming younger in mind, heart and body. It goes a long way in keeping the years off and aging well.

So whatever makes you happy, do some of that every day. Also, plan those great vacations. Nothing is more exciting than visiting another country and doing things you've never done before. Get out of your comfort zone and live a little. Repel down that 200 foot waterfall or go on a seven day bike ride in Europe or hike up a mountain and take in the view. Just get out and play a little. You won't regret it!

And as Forrest Gump said: *"That's all I have to say about that."*

Chapter 8 – The sun is not all that bad for you (did I just say that)?

Yes, I did just say that. So, what does that mean exactly? It means that hiding away from the sun is not a good idea (contrary to popular belief) and we are creating a generation of people who are vitamin D3 deficient. Check out this article from www.mindbodygreen.com called *10 Healing Benefits of the Sun* By Marcus Julian Felicetti at: https://www.mindbodygreen.com/0-5999/10-Healing-Benefits-of-the-Sun.html. This article says a lot about the need to soak in the sun. Now what I do is put on a natural sun screen that I get from a natural store – not the kind of sunscreens that are loaded with toxic chemicals that bake into your skin – and I typically will apply sunscreen to my face, neck and usually my hands if I'm getting too much sun (spending more than twenty minutes in it). This allows me to soak in the sun from other body parts.

I have to admit it's harder to get enough sun in the winter months but I do my best to get some sun exposure. In the spring, summer and most of the fall I'm typically in shorts and short sleeves. If I'm in the sun for only twenty minutes at a time with a good amount of no-exposure to the sun in between, then I don't wear any sunblock.

I realize that a lot of us don't have the option to wear whatever we want and if we are in an office environment we may be wearing suits and dresses. I would just do your best to roll up the sleeves and get outside during your lunch period and soak in some rays.

The reason why I put sunscreen on my face, neck and hands (if in the sun more than twenty minutes) is that the skin in those areas are very sensitive and it is always exposed (at least for most of us). The face, neck and hands typically get much more sun than other body parts that are typically covered with clothing.

Another benefit of soaking in the sun is to put you in a better state of mental health. A great article from Healthline can be found here: *What Are the Benefits of Sunlight?* http://www.healthline.com/health/depression/benefits-sunlight#overview1.

This article states that both sunlight and nighttime work together to release two different hormones in your brain. Serotonin (sunlight) and Melatonin (nighttime). Serotonin will help with boosting mood and making you feel better. Melatonin will help you sleep. The two hormones work well to keep your mental and physical state in balance.

The Healthline article also goes into other benefits of the sun. Basically about twenty minutes of sun exposure a day is healthy. If you do more than that then you probably want to use sunscreen, but I recommend the most organic or natural version you can find. Whole Foods Market and other organic markets will have offerings. I would also use one that protects you from UVA and UVB and at least 30 SPF.

Now if you are going to lay out in the sun at a beach all day long I would recommend using sunscreen everywhere. Make sure to take breaks and make sure a good part of the day is under shade. Otherwise you take a chance of looking like a lobster and that's not good!

Another helpful video on www.youtube.com is from www.sunwarrior.com called *Proper Exposure: Benefits of Sunlight | Dr. Weston* at https://www.youtube.com/watch?v=GJsprD5bO70.

This video discusses the importance of getting some sun exposure. It's crazy that we always seem to go from one extreme to the other of an argument without stopping in the middle. We went from getting too much sun decades ago to getting no sun today. Why wouldn't we think about stopping somewhere in the middle of these two extremes? Why are we scared of something that life would be impossible without? Anyway, these are some of the topics in Dr. Weston's video. Please take a look.

This was a very short chapter but a very important one. I know there is so much conflicting information out there and it's hard to decide what to do but I would recommend not hiding from the sun. It has, after all, been in our world since the beginning and we wouldn't exist without it. What I'm saying is common sense should and will always prevail. A little sun every day is good. Too much exposure is not. I guess the same can be said for red wine and dark chocolate!

Chapter 9 – Other little tips

So, you are doing all the other stuff that I recommended: eating organically, gluten and dairy free, drinking plenty of water (probably the most important single thing you can do), doing your hair massages, doing your face massages and exercises, working out with aerobic and resistance training, meditating and keeping a positive mental outlook and getting your necessary sun exposure (not over exposure) but you want to do more?

Really?

Okay, here are a few more tips before you finish the book. Some of these are going to be common sense, but here goes:

Sleeping:

I know you have heard this many times, but the average adult should get approximately seven-and-a-half to eight hours of sleep every night. I know this is hard to do for most of us but you should do your best to do this consistently. A good article on sleep is found in the WebMD article: *Sleep through the decades - How sleep changes with age, once you're an adult by Gina Shaw:* http://www.webmd.com/sleep-disorders/features/adult-sleep-needs-and-habits#1.

From this article, you will see that we are, on average, sleeping about one hour less than average adults in the 1960's and 1970's. The world is a lot faster now and because of it most of us don't get enough sleep at night. Do your best to get your sleep because it can keep you healthy, fresh and feeling and looking younger.

I hear people complain that they have a hard time falling asleep or having quality sleep. One thing I noticed that if I'm watching TV or surfing the web with my tablet or phone while in bed, it disrupts my ability to get a good night's sleep. If you are in that pattern, try to break out of it and put those devices away. Turn the TV off and just try to relax. A list of twenty good points to help can be found in this WebMD article: *20 tips for better sleep -Reviewed by William Blahd, MD :* http://www.webmd.com/a-to-z-guides/discomfort-15/better-sleep/slideshow-sleep-tips. Give some of these great tips a try and I'm sure you will get better sleep, feel better during the day and start to look and feel years younger.

One of my favorite tips in this article is to wake up and go to sleep about the same time every day and night respectively. This helps to get the body into a pattern. I have to admit I don't follow this all the time since there are going to be circumstances where I'm out late at a concert, or event, or up early for a special event, but I do follow it the best I can (that's a common theme of mine, isn't it)?

Here is another good article from WebMD that discusses the benefits of getting the right amount of sleep: *Beauty Sleep: 5 tips for your skin - By Stephanie Booth, Reviewed by Carol DerSarkissian:*

. The first bullet point goes into how sleep can help you look younger by promoting cell and tissue repair. Sleep also helps your body's ability to produce new collagen that keeps skin healthy and elastic.

So, in summary, make sure you are getting your sleep in. Again, the average adult should get approximately eight hours of sleep at night so if you are well below or above this number you might want to rethink your sleep patterns.

<u>Nice Trick to help Whiten Teeth</u>:

There are a few ways to help whiten teeth naturally and I'm going to bring up two of them that I tried and experienced positive results. The first one involves coconut oil.   This video from the Dr. Oz show demonstrates how it is done: *Natural Teeth Whitening Solutions:* .
Basically, you put a teaspoon of coconut oil (it will be solid at room temperature) in your mouth (the coconut oil will melt) and swish it around for about 20 minutes or so (yes this is a long time and you may want to start at a few minutes and then build up to the 20). The oil will liquefy due to the heat of your body. You will need to spit it out when you are done because the coconut oil will pull (remove) toxins and bacteria from your mouth and teeth and you don't want to swallow that garbage. I attempt to do this every day but I realistically average one to two times a week – and not always make the full 20 minutes.

Another good way to whiten teeth naturally is with lemon juice and baking soda. You can find the procedure in this article on the Every Day Roots website (www.everydayroots.com) at: *3 Natural Ways to Whiten Teeth at Home:* http://everydayroots.com/teeth-whitening-at-home. Basically, you mix a teaspoon of baking soda with a little lemon juice. The mixture will fizz up and you can mix it while it's fizzing. Once it stops fizzing you will see a pasty type product. Use it to brush your teeth as you would with regular tooth paste. Then rinse. I try to do this once per week, no more. It doesn't taste great but it's over quickly.

Lotion, face creams, etc.

Maybe because I'm a guy I haven't dabbled much in face creams. With that said I do use a very natural, non-scented lotion for face, neck, hands and body. I get mine from Whole Foods and it works well. I do use it all over my body and I put it on right after I shower and on my face, neck and hands before going to bed. I also will apply a natural sun screen on my face, neck and hands only if I'm going to be in the sun for more than 20 minutes a day. I use 30 SPF and make sure it protects for UVA & UVB. I leave the rest of my body exposed to the sun so I can get the vitamin D3 benefit. If I am going to be sunbathing at a beach for the day, I will use sunscreen over the rest of my body and take sun breaks. Otherwise I would burn. Some sun exposure is good but too much – not so good! For more on sun exposure see *Chapter 8 – The sun is not all that bad for you (did I just say that)?*

My main point here is to try to treat your skin like you treat the rest of your body (after all it's the largest organ of your body). You want to nourish it with lotion but you don't want all the chemicals, artificial dyes or scents. Remember that lotion is absorbed by the skin and enters your body so, go to a natural organic store to get your lotions as well.

Removing Age Spots:

In scanning the Internet I've come across a lot of remedies for removing age spots. The one that I've tried and works for me is using lemon juice twice a day. It takes about six weeks to see results and you have to do it consistently every day. There is an article from Organic Facts (www.organicfacts.com) at: *How To Get Rid Of Brown Spots On Skin: http://www.top10homeremedies.com/how-to/how-to-get-rid-of-brown-spots-on-skin.html.* That article discusses the lemon juice as well as other methods to rid of age spots. I can't speak for the other methods mentioned in this article because I didn't try them yet, but I will state that I've seen good results from the lemon juice method.

I do use an oil based application that I mentioned in *Chapter 3 – Yes, you can really grow back your hair!* I'll repost that information in italics below so you can skip it if you already read it (I used this oil concoction for my scalp and hair as well as my face, neck and hands:

Another good video on a hair oil can be found on EricTipsReviews! (https://www.youtube.com/channel/UCEP2Salwz1kLMp292iOfW_w) at: Grow THICKER HAIR NATURALLY with oils!!!! (https://www.youtube.com/watch?v=1v2PRuxoMp8). Eric's recipe ncorporates six different oils and each oil brings something to facilitate hair growth. I've made this recipe and I have to say I'm very happy with t. The oils he uses are: coconut, Emu, jojoba, sweet almond, caster & vitamin E. I've also made this recipe but replaced the Emu oil with olive oil. Partly because I like the benefits olive oil brings to the table and I feel a little bad for the Emus that give up their lives just for the oil. I also put n a few drops of peppermint oil and frankincense oil. I would definitely recommend you giving this concoction or the many others in youtube (www.youtube.com) a try!

Soap, shampoo, lotions, etc.

I'm not going to spend too much time here but I will touch on it. When I shower I use a natural/organic soap that I find at my local health food store. I make sure to get one that has no dyes and is unscented, because I don't want to smell like a flower, but if you want all that, there are lots of options for natural/organic soap with natural fragrance and color.

My reasoning behind using natural/organic soap is that I want to treat the outside of my body the same way I treat the inside. So, if I'm not going to consume a bunch of chemicals I'm also going to try not to smear them all over my body as well. Now if I'm out and about and I use a public restroom (or at a friend's house) or I'm travelling, I'll go ahead and use their soap. I'm not fanatic enough yet to carry my own soap but who knows what the future holds for me.

As for shampoo and conditioner, I try not to use shampoo more than once or twice a week. That statement in the past would have surprised my wife and son because they know that I used to shampoo and condition my hair every time I took a shower. And because of the exercising I do, I typically shower two to three times a day so, yes, I used to shampoo and condition my hair that often. Unfortunately, this is not good for hair and I think it might have had a small contribution to my male-pattern baldness. So I limit the shampoo but I *condition* my hair every time I shower.

Once I read Rob's book at www.perfecthairhealth.com, I learned that it was unnecessary to wash my hair that frequently. In fact, I believe Rob seldom washes his hair with shampoo and relies mainly on water to do the job. When I do use shampoo and conditioner I make sure to use an organic/natural one that I get at a health food store. Again, just making sure I keep the chemicals at bay. You may hear that sulfates are harsh on hair and it's in most shampoos. Go ahead and look at the ingredients on the label and you will see. Stay away from the sulfates!

A great, and funny, video regarding sulfates in shampoos can be found on Youtube from Penny Tovar (https://www.youtube.com/channel/UCD0XqR_pfjolXudnjkeHglw) at: *How to Check Shampoo for Sulfates:* https://www.youtube.com/watch?v=XUwQxMuYpv0. She's a little silly but gives a helpful list of chemicals to look for in your shampoo. If yours has one or more of these sulfates you may want to change your shampoo!

After I shower I do use lotion all over my body. You guessed it, I use an organic/natural one with no scent and no artificial colors.

Antiperspirant vs. deodorant:

Some people would recommend not using either but hey, we live in a civilized society and we owe it to our fellow man, woman & child to keep our own body odor at bay. I would suggest a good natural/organic unscented deodorant (not antiperspirant) that you can find at your local health food store. Why do I not recommend antiperspirant? First you have to know the difference between the two. Antiperspirant stops you from sweating and blocks odor. Deodorant blocks odor but lets you sweat. The body was meant to sweat so to stop it is not a good idea. So I recommend staying away from the antiperspirant and going with the natural or organic deodorant.

Enough is enough!

Ok, I think between the scalp massages, facial massages and exercises, body exercises, getting your mind right, nutrition changes, getting more sun, whitening your teeth, getting enough sleep, drinking more water, reducing age spots and other aging well techniques, that you probably have more than enough to start working on so I'm going to stop here. I would recommend picking just a couple of changes to your life at first and when you get those under control to move on to others. If you try to take on everything at the same time you will, more than likely, lose your mind and quit. Good luck with all of this and try your very best to have fun on your journey to the fountain of youth. If you can enjoy your journey and continue it for the rest of your life, you will, more than likely, look and feel years younger!

Chapter 10 – The story of my life (basically about the author)

So, you want to know a little about me? Well here goes. I was born in 1961 and lived in the suburbs of Washington, DC in the great state of Maryland. I was always a skinny kid and even though I wanted to play football in high school, Seneca Valley – go Eagles, they wouldn't allow a 115-pound adolescent on the team. I wasn't happy but understood. That was a lawsuit waiting to happen!

I wanted to do something with sports so I did what all the skinny teenagers did. I joined the Cross-Country team. I learned a lot about teamwork, hard work and a lot about being healthy. I also ran track.

I attended the University of Maryland, College Park – go Terps! I wasn't good enough to be on a Division 1 cross country and track team but I continued running. It was around my junior year where I started lifting weights as well and thought more about what I put in my mouth. It was then when I quit drinking sodas completely and reduced the amount of processed sugar in my diet.

After graduating from college with a Bachelor's of Science in business, majoring in accounting, and spending six months down in Florida, I came back to Maryland and started my first job as an accountant at a small biotech firm. After three years, I took and passed the Certified Public Accountant (CPA) exam and moved my professional career to the headquarters of the American Red Cross. That's where I met my wife and moved up the corporate ladder to become Sr. Director of Financial Management. My wife gave birth to our only child, Matt, and after a seventeen year career with the American Red Cross my wife and I decided to start a business near our house so we could spend more time with our son (we were losing two to three hours a day commuting) and get back a big part of our lives.

We opened a Fleet Feet specialty running store (it's a franchise) and had a great thirteen year run until we decided to go into semi-retirement and, at the time of this publication, purchased a house in sunny California near the beach in San Diego County. We wanted to spend more time outdoors in the perfect weather north of San Diego (after all you only live once)!

During our ownership of a Fleet Feet store I was surrounded with very helpful people – customers, our staff, Fleet Feet Inc. staff, other Fleet Feet owners and staff, our great vendor reps and support teams and the owners of the other fantastic local businesses in our area. I learned a lot about exercising and healthy eating. That's when I went nearly 100% organic, had a great time running with our customers and found out about the workouts on www.beachbody.com.

On the side I also wrote my novel, *Memoirs of Biochip Man*, which can be found on www.amazon.com at https://www.amazon.com/Christopher-Welch-

Life was going well but then I noticed I was losing my hair fast so I looked at every remedy out there. I did start Minoxidil and it helped a little but I didn't like spreading chemicals all over my scalp. Eventually I came across Rob's book at www.perfecthairhealth.com and started his recommendations.   From there, and still exploring the Internet, I came across Patricia Goroway's video on facial health which you can find here: *Facial Fitness System by Patricia Goroway:* at: https://www.youtube.com/watch?v=0diJ1hx4lbI&list=PLnvpR2oTa8rlMLf 5cZ5lvHQ0cEr3AiLbE and Olgatoja for facial massage at: https://www.youtube.com/user/olgatoja. From there I found other great videos and articles that helped with my facial health.

When my hair started to grow back and I saw lines fade from my face, as well as keeping my body in great shape, I thought that others would benefit from the same information I possessed so I wrote this book, created a website (www.christophergault.com) and www.youtube.com channel at: https://www.youtube.com/channel/UCaWrxHvVbEinWXUPwno9k3A?vie w_as=subscriber. Hopefully these tools will help you as well to obtain your goal of looking and feeling years younger.

Chapter 11 – Necessary disclaimer

This book contains information that should *not* be considered as medical advice and *not* be used in lieu of a qualified doctor to diagnose or treat any health problems. If you do have health problems, I recommend seeing your doctor for it.

If the reader chooses to implement any of these lifestyle changes recommended in this book, they must do so with the understanding they are fully responsible for their actions.

Applying the information contained in this book is at the sole risk and choice of the reader.

The author and affiliates are not responsible for damages caused to the reader as a result of the information or recommendations presented within this book.

Chapter 12 – Copyright

This Book is meant to act as a guide to help you gain your youthful appearance and health. This Book highlights my experience utilizing information found on the Internet. It does not guarantee that you will achieve the same results as the author.

The information in this Book does not replace any medical, legal, or professional advice. Please use this information at your own risk. And above all, consult your doctor if you have any questions or concerns about the recommendations in this book.

Chapter 13 – Conclusion (my last thoughts)

So, you finished the book! Either that or you skipped ahead to see the conclusion before reading the book. Either way just picking this book up could be the start of your journey to the fountain of youth and to look and feel years younger.

I wish I could say I am an expert in health and looking and feeling years younger but I'm not. I'm just an average person who doesn't want to accept that we all have to fall apart when we age. I don't want to accept that I have to see muscle loss, the skin on my face slipping off and going bald. It was actually going bald that started me on my trip down the Internet in the first place. I was losing my hair a lot faster than my friends and family members and I could have either accepted that fate or I could change it. Once I started down that road I found that there was more than just hair that I wasn't happy with as I aged.

One thing I also gained on my journey was I realized that I really was in control of my life. Not just for aging well but in all aspects of it. I didn't like my commute to work, so I changed that by opening up my own business a mile from my house. I always wanted to live on the west coast so I am moving there shortly. This journey really helped me take control of the reigns of my life and I am still taking control to this day. Where it will lead me, who knows. I strongly recommend everyone take responsibility and control over their own lives. Once you do you will feel great, trust me!

I was always in pretty good shape because I've always worked out in my teen and adult life. There were times when I felt like stopping but seeing others that were even younger than me let themselves go, I knew I didn't want to become like that. To have several pounds more on me than I should was not an option and I saw what happens to people when they have horrible diets. You can see the effects on their skin and their bodies. It's sad. I also don't want to get to the point where I'm bent over so far that I'm looking at the street while I'm walking with my cane or walker.

So, I decided to take on age head-on and reverse the process the best way I could. I also felt a need to share my journey with the rest of the world in the hopes that others would feel the same way I do and take control of their own lives and change them in a positive way.

Since you picked up this book it sounds as if you are one of these people. Please take on these exercises and procedures, do them consistently, have patience and wait for the results and you will be grateful you did. Because if you can pull off what is in this book and keep it going for ten months to a year, you, your friends and family members, will be amazed at the transformation. You will also learn to love life more and be happy.

I can't finish the book without stating the following: I am not a big fan of the term *anti-aging*. It implies that you don't age anymore which basically means you're dead, or trapped in space.   I prefer the term *aging well*. This implies that you are still breathing, which is a good thing, but you are slowing down the effects of aging. Basically you are staying physically and mentally strong and living the best life you can. Living the dream! Because, as we all know, you only live once, so why not make it the best possible life!

One last note, if you have any comments and/or questions, please go to my website at www.christopher.com, my youtube channel at: https://www.youtube.com/channel/UCaWrxHvVbEinWXUPwno9k3A?view_as=subscriber,   or   my   facebook   page   at: https://www.facebook.com/Gault-Author-Page-407815659707073   and send them to me. I can't promise but I will try to respond to all comments and questions I receive.

So, good luck on your journey and I hope the best!

www.ingramcontent.com/pod-product-compliance
Lightning Source LLC
Chambersburg PA
CBHW051352280526
45784CB00007B/2926